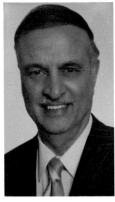

Dr. Dinker Rai I Chairman of the Department of Surgery, as the Chief of the Department of Vascular Surgery/Vascular Laboratory at the Interfaith Medical Center, Brooklyn, New York. A Visiting associate clinical professor at State Univ. of NY, Brooklyn and visiting Professor of surgery at Rajiv Gandhi Univ Bangalore, India.

He invented the first ever method for retrograde catheterization of the venous tree and was given a US patent. Based on this patent, The Ideas For Medicine, Inc. (now part of Horizon Medical Products, Inc.) manufactured and distributes out a series of Rai's Catheters for use in performing descending phlebography and for venous embolectomies. Dr. Rai has a series of discoveries. The first one is motion of venous valves in human beings. almost 500 years after Fabricus Acquapedente of Padua Univ discovered function of the venous valves. He discovered that venous blood flow is pulsatile which, prior to this was described only as linear flow. His original research on histopathological specimens of patients with saphenofemoral – incompetency resulted in a paradigm shift in management of varicose veins. He performed the first ever vein valve transplantation below the knee. His monumental work is the discovery of right atrial mechanical function is a pivotal discovery in his medical research field. He has authored two chapters in textbook of Angiology and wrote a beginner's manual on sclerotherapy and management of varicose veins with stab phlebectomy. He conducted many workshops across the world to popularize this treatment for varicose veins and is a pioneer in the field of venous surgery with several publications and presentations.

He is an accomplished Artist and can notice in this book. At age 14, a portrait he made of then US President John F. Kennedy, was presented to President who reciprocated with letter of appreciation. At present, preserved and exhibited at JFK library in Boston.

Dr. Rai was an accomplished sportsman and captained the Bangalore University cricket team winning the south zone. He captained the Combined Universities Cricket team of the South hb Zone of India and Sri Lanka in 1969. when selected for the Karnataka Ranji team in 1970 opted mecicine over cricket. In lieu of his contribution to cricket, his name is on the Honor Roll at the Chinnaswamy Stadium Cricket Museum in Bangalore.

Dr. Rai has a keen interest in philosophy. A student of Sanskrit. He has contributed many articles on various subjects and published in Bhavan's and other reputed Journals. He served as the Chairman of the Bharatiya Vidya Bhavan, United States.

Dinker B. Rai, MD

Mechanical Function of the Atrial Diastole

Mechanical Function of the Atrial Diastole: A New Discovery

The Motion of Blood in the Venous System—Novel Findings

Dinker B. Rai, MD

Past Chairman, Department of Surgery
Chief, Department of Vascular Surgery/Vascular Laboratory
Interfaith Medical Center
Brooklyn, New York, USA

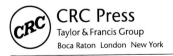

CRC Press
Taylor & Francis Group
Boca Raton London New York

CRC Press is an imprint of the
Taylor & Francis Group, an **informa** business

First edition published 2022
by CRC Press
6000 Broken Sound Parkway NW, Suite 300, Boca Raton, FL 33487-2742

and by CRC Press
2 Park Square, Milton Park, Abingdon, Oxon, OX14 4RN

CRC Press is an imprint of Taylor & Francis Group, LLC

© 2022 Taylor & Francis Group, LLC

Library of Congress Cataloging-in-Publication Data

Names: Rai, Dinker B., author.
Title: Mechanical function of the atrial diastole : a new discovery and the motion of blood in the venous system-novel findings / Dinker B. Rai.
Description: First edition. | Boca Raton : CRC Press, 2022. | Includes bibliographical references and index.
Identifiers: LCCN 2021045290 (print) | LCCN 2021045291 (ebook) | ISBN 9781032198477 (hardback) | ISBN 9781032209371 (paperback) | ISBN 9781003266006 (ebook)
Subjects: MESH: Blood Circulation--physiology | Venous Pressure--physiology | Atrial Function--physiology | Pulsatile Flow--physiology
Classification: LCC QP101 (print) | LCC QP101 (ebook) | NLM WG 103 | DDC 612.1/3--dc23
LC record available at https://lccn.loc.gov/2021045290
LC ebook record available at https://lccn.loc.gov/2021045291

ISBN: 978-1-032-19847-7 (hbk)
ISBN: 978-1-032-20937-1 (pbk)
ISBN: 978-1-003-26600-6 (ebk)

DOI: 10.1201/b22792

Typeset in Palatino LT Std
by KnowledgeWorks Global Ltd.

Printed in the UK by Severn, Gloucester on responsibly sourced paper

Contents

Preface.. vii
Foreword by Seshadri Raju... xiii
Foreword by Kailash Prasad xvii
Prologue... xxi

Chapter 1   The history of circulation 1
Phases of the history of circulation 1
The theory of circulation—pre-Galenic era 1
The theory of circulation—Galenic era 4
Historical impact..8

Chapter 2   Sir William Harvey....................................11
Background... 11
Methods...12
Experimental revelation of Sir William Harvey..........14
The next great discovery..15
Theory of circulation by Sir William Harvey 19

Chapter 3   Present concept 23

Chapter 4   Mystery of the venous valves 27
History..29

Chapter 5   Motion of blood in the venous
            system—novel findings 31
Velocity—a new parameter 31
Objective..34
Materials..34
Method..35

Findings..38
Discussion...41
Conclusion...42

Chapter 6   Venous flow is pulsatile........................**45**
Method...47

Chapter 7   Motion of venous valves in
 humans—a new discovery........................**51**
History of modern medicine.....................................51
Management of venous disorders............................52
Author's personal experience...................................52
Methods..53
Results..54
Discussion...55
Conclusion...58
Author's reflection...58

Chapter 8   The dynamic function of the
 atrial diastole of the heart........................**61**
Description...63
Study on canines..63
Discussion...70
Conclusion...73

Chapter 9   Theory of circulation by the author........**75**
Concepts of the circulatory system.........................75
Classification of circulation......................................77
New insights..79

References..83
Index...85

Preface

"VAKRA THUNDA MAHAKAYA KOTI SURYA SAMAPRABHA
NIRVIGNAM KURUME DEVA SARVA KARYESHU SARVADHA"

("Broken tusked, humongous bodied, radiating the effulgence
equal to tens of millions of simultaneously dazzling suns in
the sky. Oh! Lord clear the obstacles in all my undertakings all
the time")

In the voyage of life, we all walk through an unwritten path. Only
the stretch I trodden heretofore I can recollect and contemplate
upon. The most difficult gaps of my path where I lost myself, I
now see were made up of bridges to overcome and reach the other
side. There were different bridges to cover different aspects of life,
but in achieving this monumental work of my life in my medical
career the whole path appears like one long bridge. The pillars that
held the bridge for me to cross were held by some very important
people or institutions and books of information and sometimes
rare resources who came and passed across in my life for what
reason I cannot fathom. Many a time, I felt they were specifically
picked for the sole purpose to help me out in difficult situations.

There is nothing I can do to repay their service. The comple-
tion of my work and bringing it out in the form of a book, it is
time for me to acknowledge and pay my tribute to those who
played the role of the pillars for me to cross the bridge. First, I
have to thank the institution, Brooklyn Jewish Medical Center,
where I began my first day of surgical internship and continue to
work still to this day in the same department. Apart from being
the most reputed hospital and the earliest one in the Borough of
Brooklyn, it also had a tradition for being an educational center

with active research going on. It had a monkey and a canine lab which is a luxury for any researcher to have in his own institution. Many internationally recognized, groundbreaking discoveries were made, and I inherited that legacy. As a resident, my exposure to these labs and dissecting canines helped me to conduct my experimental work. Later, when I became an attending in surgery, I had the canine lab at my disposal. I was free to work any time and any day of the week. Almost always, most of the research work is carried out by those in the faculties. Therefore, being an actively practicing surgeon, it was very handy for me to work in the lab during my free time. It was all made easy because of the help I received from Dr. Robert Lerner who was the Chairman of Surgery at that time. He had immense faith in my work, which boosted my self-confidence and warded off my doubts. He obtained help for me from various departments and whenever I needed it. That is the main reason why I was able to do and contribute in areas other than my own field of vascular surgery, such as diagnostic radiology, nuclear radiology, pathology and physiology. It included new inventions, creation of diagnostic and therapeutic procedures, inventing new catheters to perform the same tasks with a USA patent, and new surgical procedures and discoveries.

I thank pathologist Dr. Shamah Iqbal who helped me dissect and harvest venous valves from cadavers. Both of us first studied the histology of varicose veins and gave the first ever description of it in the history of histopathology. I thank Dr. Vandana Chokshi, Chief of Nuclear Radiology, to accept my novel concept of venous velocity and developing a model to study with nuclear radiology methods and the development of a time velocity curve. Both of them had to sacrifice their free time to accommodate me.

Most of my work was done late evening or weekends when I was free of my regular commitments of patient care and private practice. All of my work in the canine lab was conducted on weekends. It used to be long hours of dissection of canine models before starting any experimental work. I started in the early morning and ended late in the evening. I thank two of the surgical residents who helped me immensely by assisting in dissections and voluntarily participating in these experiments and providing me with timely and worthy suggestions. It is but for their selfless help the job would have been hardly possible to complete. I thank

Dr. Indrajlt Singh and Dr. Carlos Ortego, as they too sacrificed time being in a grueling surgical residency program.

The second part of my journey is of a greater ordeal of collection of data and interpretation in order to put various pieces of the puzzle into the right place. Atrial diastole was always thought to be an inactive functionless phenomenon. Atrial chambers were not even considered an anatomical component of the human heart from the beginning and extending to a period even after the time of Sir William Harvey and his new discoveries. This was the stopping block to me. Every time I made thoughtful experiments and any progress it would ultimately come to a halt there. So, my quest continued to find an answer lasted several years. I desperately tried to obtain help from any source possible. I explored all the past history on this subject and looked into the ancient countries and their practice of medicine, including Egyptian, Assyrian, Babylonian, Hebrew medicine mostly based on the old and new testaments, Japanese and Chinese who practiced the WU medicine, and Greek medicine as popularized later by Galen. Nowhere was the human heart given any importance as the organ of circulation. Assyrian, Babylonian and Greek medicine provided great importance to the liver as the main organ of circulation, and most likely due to the fact that it lies in the middle of the human body, is large and it is filled with blood.

Indian scriptures and sciences of Yoga and Ayurveda provided great importance to the human heart. From an unknown time, they considered the heart the most important organ of the human body giving it sacred and physical importance. They named it HRIDAYA, which appears like the root word of HEART. Thousands of years earlier, Lord Krishna mentioned this organ even in his recitation of Bhagavat Geetha the holy book of Hindus and is noteworthy. There must have been genuine reason it was considered the main organ of the human body in that part of ancient world culture and science. Doctrines of Galen gave the utmost importance to the liver probably because he noticed it as a large organ lying at the midway of the body absorbing all the nutrition from the intestines and spreading it to the rest of the body. This is explained in more in detail in the subsequent chapters of the book. Ayurveda medical science of ancient India provided detailed descriptions of human heart. These were mostly lost in the books written in the Sanskrit language. Most of this science was systematically destroyed over time as the historical changes took place in the country. As the dust of time settled, the remnants if any, left over in the treatises of Charaka and Sushrutha were the only available material, and even that may not be complete work. To lay hands on this, it was necessary for me to learn the Sanskrit language. I had a timely teacher, Dr. P. Jayaraman, a great scholar of Sanskrit. He was patient enough to teach me the language and introduce me to abundant Sanskrit literature. He translated for me the available remnants of Shushrutha Sahmitha written by the great Indian surgeon Shushruta. Historically more than 80% of that literature has been destroyed. During this time, he also introduced me to other Sanskrit literature of interest, including the great works of Kalidasa and various Upanishads. What attracted my attention and opened my mind the most was the opening verse (Sloka) of "Isha Vasya Upanishad," whose meaning is "Universe is the Abode of the Lord." In the very opening sentence at the outset Sage declares, coining the word "Jagath" to describe the universe. He phrases it as "Jagathyam Jagath." He coins the noun Jagath on the basis of the adjective Jagathyam, which reveals the secret of universe itself, and that is, it is a phenomenon continuously in a state of motion resulting continuous change and it is the unsurpassable law of the universe. This enlightened an exciting spot in my mind, splashing the corollary of the truth that both the atria and ventricle are bound by the same law because they very much form the components of the universe. When a motion is changed in the human body at specific junctures, it may give a feeling of comfort to the mind. So, the word "REST" was created to represent a passive, non-functional state of motion and is a myth which does not exist. It was created to express a feeling of comfort. The word REST is an imaginary creation of the human mind. It convinced me the human heart is no exception, whether ventricles or the atrium are both bound by the laws of the universal phenomenon of existence. Both diastole and systole are active events which carry their own function. In addition, both diastole and systole are accompanied by physical, chemical and electrical changes at the cellular level. Once this was clear, I was able to decipher the graphic curves and the atrial diastolic function was revealed to me. The remainder of the components of the puzzle fell into their proper place once the main puzzle was solved.

My last mission was to publish the experimental findings of atrial diastolic function in a peer reviewed and reputed journal. It took long time and I was met with many rejections before this new concept was accepted, most likely due to the amount of revolutionary change. During this time, Dr. Kailash Prasad, MBBS(Hon), MD, PhD, DSc, Professor Emeritus, Department of Physiology, College of Medicine, University of Saskatchewan, Saskatoon, Canada, provided guidance and help to revise the manuscript to conform to the guidelines of a scientific journal. I thank him for the same. Ultimately, it saw the light of publication in *International Journal of Angiology*, the official journal of the International College of Angiology, in the year 2013:22;37-44.

My final responsibility was to put together all the experimental work I did pertaining to the area of hemodynamics in the form of a book. I recorded everything and I needed professional help. I thank Denise M. Rossignol, Executive Director of the International College of Angiology and Managing Editor, *International Journal of Angiology*, for giving her valuable time and energy to complete this work. She went through each sentence by sentence, correcting typographic and grammatical errors, finding references and citations, inserting diagrams at the proper places, dividing into appropriate chapters and giving my recordings a book form.

There are my family members I am indebted to for making all this journey happen in my life. My father, Kedambadi Narayana Rai a celebrated criminal lawyer of his generation. He always remains as my role model and inspired me when he was alive and continues to do so even now. At the age of 40 he suffered an acute cardiac ailment. Not well established at the time in medical science and generally called by the folk word "heart attack." The etiology or an exact treatment was unknown at that time. The only treatment I saw him receive was the compression of hot water bag, pain medications and bed rest. He suffered 7 more such attacks over the next 12 years and succumbed to the last one. A very inspiring fact to me is that he kept working and attending court until the last day of his final attack. Later, part of his ailment he used to get frequent episodes of shortness of breath during the night due to pulmonary edema. It is now very clear to me, that during these attacks his atria suffered recurrent infarctions with fibrous tissue formation losing a functioning part of the wall, and his diastolic function progressively failed causing atrial failure.

A new entity, even to this day, is not addressed. Even now, it is named as right or left heart failure which mainly addresses ventricular failure. Atrial failure in the heart is a separate entity and cannot be conceived as it is not as yet assigned a function. I thank my mother, Belle Sanjivi Rai, to stand the ordeal of the ailment of my Dad, and after the passage of my father, she held the family together and guided us as single mother. Ironically, I ended up doing research on the human heart, while not planned, but retrospectively as consolation to the suffering my parents went through caused by the heart.

It would not have been possible for me to achieve this lifetime work without the support of my wife, Mrs. Shakila Rai, who let me take precious family time and use it on research work. Right from the days of my surgical residency and later in my professional life, she gave me non-disgruntled and unconditional support. I owe her my immense gratitude.

Lastly, I thank all my teachers and students who came in my life and inspired me.

Dinker B. Rai
"Maatra Kripa"
219 Glen Cove Road
Old Westbury, New York 11568

Foreword by Seshadri Raju

Dr. Dinker Rai received his medical education in India. The political climate in India had turned hostile to professionals at that time with little chance for modern practice or advancement. In contrast, America was welcoming with open arms prompting a wave of immigration (including this writer). Dr. Rai's book opens with the sentence "I arrived in Brooklyn, New York on July 15, 1973." The *arrival* date is firmly imprinted in the mind of many a grateful immigrant to this great country, to be told and retold on countless occasions. Mine is Dec. 29, 1967. Most who came with that wave had their dreams fulfilled, many would say, beyond their wildest dreams. The material conveniences of a modern society were easy to see, but something more fundamental realized over time was unique. You were being valued for *what* you are, not *who* you are. Almost everywhere else on this globe, 'connections' of family, or those of political, religious or ethnic nature are the tickets (often fortified with bribes) to advancement. Not in this fair land, an astonishing outlier. "God Bless America" is deeply felt if not loudly spelt.

Dr. Rai started his training in general and vascular surgery at the Brooklyn Jewish Hospital (renamed Interfaith Hospital after a merger). His hard work and talents were easy to recognize. After a series of promotions, he was named to his current position as Chairman, Department of Surgery and Chief, Department of Vascular Surgery. Dr. Rai credits mentors and collaborators of diverse faiths in the hospital for his professional success. Dr. Robert Lerner receives special mention as a guide and mentor. Dr. Rai has been a leader in venous surgery which saw a renaissance in the 80's due to the enthusiasm of surgeons like him. An innovator, Dr. Rai has pioneered several important techniques and procedures. He was among the first to perform a popliteal vein valve transplantation. The ingenuity and pioneering efforts of innumerable immigrants like him have propelled the ascendancy of this country in science and technology.

The book is a hybrid product, part memoir, part medical history, but mostly about his insights in his field of venous surgery. Some of this work has been previously published, others are validated only partially, and a few more are mere kernels for development by others. The center of attention is the author's concept of atrial function which was thrust on his consciousness in an accidental way. While performing a venogram on a patient in the erect position, the table froze suddenly with the fluoroscopy still going. Struggling to hold on to the patient to prevent a fall, Dr. Rai noticed that the venous valves in the femoral vein outlined by contrast were opening and closing rhythmically. Such motion has never been described before. It set the author on a life-long quest for an explanation. It did not come easily. But the search continued, sometimes at a low level as a magnificent obsession, other times more desperately like a parent seeking a lost child and occasionally tending to become sublime like the quest for eternal truth. The search propelled the author to scour ancient medical works for clues. He even learnt Sanskrit, a notoriously difficult Indo-Caucasian language to read Indian texts on the subject. A hint of a solution came from reading the works of Sir William Harvey. Sir William noted in a letter to his friend Thomas Boyles that he would not have understood ventricular function without noticing the opening and closing of venous valves. That the noted valvular movement might be related to atrial *diastole* (deduced from simultaneous EKG tracings) was the proverbial light bulb turning on in Dr. Rai's head. He devotes several chapters in the book to describe the experiments he conducted underpinning the concept. This is a basic concept. If accepted, it would have an impact on circulatory physiology as large as that of Sir. William Harvey. A restless and ever curious mind, Dr. Rai is the author of several other original concepts in venous physiology such as for example, venous pulsations and venous velocity. He devotes a few chapters in the book to these. In one such chapter he gives a detailed description of measuring venous velocity in iliac veins. Venous practioners will appreciate the detailed description of diagnostic techniques such as descending venography and surgical procedures to address superficial or chronic deep venous disease. Dr. Rai has a holistic understanding of venous disease. At this level, it is no longer rote science, but pure art. If asked to explain, the master is often unable, as it is not divisible into parts. It is astonishing to learn that Dr. Rai has been performing saphenous sparing varicose vein surgery for several decades. It is all the rage now among 'experts' for the past 10 years.

The book is eminently readable with interesting tidbits and anecdotes. For example, we learn that Sir William Harvey softened his theory of circulation to mollify adherents of Galen. Alas, to no avail, as he had to hide for two years for fear of assassination by Galen's enraged followers. The book is decorated with the author's original drawings rendered beautifully with his annotations in near calligraphic precision.

Seshadri Raju M.D., FACS
Emeritus Professor of Surgery
University of Mississippi School of Medicine
Director, The Rane Center for Venous and Lymphatic Disease

Foreword by Kailash Prasad

The book entitled *Mechanical Function of Atrial Diastole: A New Discovery—The Motion of Blood in the Venous System: Novel Findings* written by Dr. Dinker B. Rai, MD, contains 9 chapters including the history of circulation theory of Sir William Harvey, present concept, the mystery of venous valves, motion of blood in the venous system, pulsatile venous flow, motion of venous valves in humans, dynamic function of the atrial diastole, the author's concept and theory of circulation and the mystery of venous valves. The author's novel findings include, motion of blood in the venous system, pulsatile venous flow, motion of venous valves in humans, dynamic function of the atrial diastole and the concept and theory of circulation. Each section begins with a series of learning objectives. Emphasis has been laid on the important facts, topics and concepts that have been covered. The author constructed a framework to which his own concepts and theory of circulation have been added. The knowledge of physiology of circulation is cumulative with new information building on the past information. It is difficult to understand advanced material without knowing the previous concept and theory.

Dr. Rai has given the history of circulation from the era of Galen to Sir William Harvey. According to Galen, a famous philosopher/physician who lived during the 2nd century, nourishment is taken from the intestines via the portal vein and the liver transforms this nourishment into blood and distributes it to the various parts of the body. Sir William Harvey brought the actual present theory of blood circulation. His discovery on circulation shows that the heart has four chambers; right and left atria and ventricles.

Dr. Rai, a famous vascular surgeon, thought that there is a mysterious role of venous valves. He got the idea of the role of the atrium in venous circulation while performing a descending phlebography on patients. However, he felt that it is a great task to prove his idea against established concepts of circulation of blood and the laws of muscle contraction established by noble minds in the past. His experiments on canines led to a new discovery on atrial diastolic function of human heart and contributed a new concept on the motion of blood in the venous system and the laws of muscle contraction of the heart. He has described in detail the supradiaphragmatic, trans-brachial and ipsilateral vein approach to assess occlusion and valve function. This author has proved that systole and diastole are equally active phases of the cardiac cycle and contribute equally to the function of the heart. His discoveries are (1) Atrial diastole is an active phenomenon and function like a suction machine of the human heart. It keeps the blood in motion. (2) Venous blood flow is pulsatile. (3) Venous valves open and close during each cardiac cycle and is secondary to atrial diastole. (4) The function of the atrium is to keep blood in motion in the venous system. (5) Cardiac muscles contract and stretch and both are active phenomenon.

The author has made a most ambitious and formidable undertaking of compiling this book and presenting his discovery. His concept is very credible and adds to the present available concept and theory of venous circulation, venous valve movement and atrial relaxation. This book provides a comprehensive text on new concepts and basic understanding of the physiology of venous circulation which will be useful in the diagnosis and treatment of venous diseases. Furthermore, this book would be of value for basic scientists, physicians, surgeons, medical students, interns, residents and other related health professionals.

In conclusion, this new concept is a great advancement in the venous circulation, venous valve movement and relaxation of atrium. Dr. Dinker B. Rai should be congratulated for this discovery.

Kailash Prasad, BSc (Distinction),
MBBS (Hons), MD, PhD, DSc,
FRCPC, FACC, FIACS, FICA
Professor Emeritus, Department of Physiology (APP)
College of Medicine, University of Saskatchewan
Saskatoon, Saskatchewan, S7K 3Z2, Canada
&
Chairman, Board of Directors
International College of Angiology
Jay, Vermont, USA

Prologue

On July 15, 1973, I arrived in Brooklyn, New York, as a new graduate of Bangalore Medical College. I did my schooling in St. Aloysius, Mangalore, India. Upon finishing medical school, I spent two years as a tutor in Anatomy at the Kasturba Medical College in Manipal, India. I joined Brooklyn Jewish Medical Center (Brooklyn, New York) as a surgical intern under the leadership of Dr. Bernard Levowitz, who was the Chairman of the Department of Surgery, and a dynamic person dedicated to teaching and research at a 900-plus bed hospital with multi-specialties.

The Brooklyn Jewish Medical Center held a long-standing reputation for research, education and state of the art patient care, so much so, that, Albert Einstein underwent surgery for an abdominal aortic aneurysm with the first external stent performed by Dr. Rudolph Nissen in 1945. Further discoveries at Brooklyn Jewish Medical Center was the Rh blood factor, discovered in Rhesus monkeys by Landsteiner and Wiener.

Upon completing my surgical training and vascular fellowship at Maimonides Medical Center (Brooklyn, New York), I joined the staff at Brooklyn Jewish Hospital as an attending in the department of surgery. This department had a very high-powered cardiovascular department, and arterial surgery had just captured the imagination of surgeons and evolved into a new and promising field across the country. As a young new attending in vascular surgery, I was at the bottom of the ladder to compete with well-established senior surgeons to attract private referrals. Considering this, and in order to make a living, I opted to look into other areas under the vascular surgery specialty, and as a result, I ended up treating the most neglected group of patients of the time, those who were suffering from non-healing intractable ulcers secondary to chronic venous insufficiency disease (CVID). In general, those suffering from these foul-smelling ulcers, were passed down to those interns just beginning their career in the medical field.

No sooner than I began accepting and treating these patients, I started accumulating them in my office from various referrals. During this time, I provided periodic tender care with cleaning and dressing their ulcers. At that time, and under the prevailing knowledge and developments without an alternative treatment to offer. After a while, this treatment proved to be uninspiring, as there appeared to be an improvement to the condition of the disease. It was this factor which motivated me to pursue in depth, the venous system from a different perspective, where lies the etiology of venous ulcers.

Coincidentally, Dr. Robert Kistner performed the first ever femoral vein valvuloplasty in 1971. This caught the interest of Dr. Sheshadri Raju of Jackson, Mississippi, a renowned cardio-thoracic surgeon, who popularized the concept of valvuloplasty. Later, a very innovative surgeon, Dr. Syed Taheri of Williamsville, New York performed the first vein valve transplantation of the femoral vein. Dr. Taheri began pioneering work on developing a prosthetic vein valve, and during the same decade, the use of sclerotherapy in the management of varicose veins had been reintroduced in a more scientific manner.

Initially, sclerotherapy was performed in isolation by few of us scattered across the country who belonged to different specialties and together we communicated and exchanged our concepts. This resulted in a desire among us to form a new platform to enhance the art and the idea of forming a society was born. Dr. Ken Biegeleisen took the lead and rejuvenated the old dormant Phlebology Society of America with a freshly elected Board of Directors, and thus I joined the group. A new hope emerged in the understanding and treatment of venous ailments. We all became the initial participants in pioneering this new movement in the country. Soon it attracted the attention of prominent vascular surgeons, dermatologists and radiologists across the nation and resulted in the formation of new societies dedicated to this field. Phlebology became a new subspecialty.

I used to perform descending phlebography on CVID patients to study the competency of the venous valves. I personally conducting these procedures in the radiology department, as it was not familiar to radiologist, and in doing so, I devised a catheter to advance in a retrogade fashion in the veins, through the venous valves without causing any damage to the veins. Upon receiving a patent for this device, ideas for Medicine a company from Tampa Fl, started producing these catheters. It is used to perform venous embolectomies as well, and all these events renewed the interest in the study of venous valves.

In 1984, this author performed the first vein valve transplant in the popliteal vein below the knee. During that same time period, while performing a descending phlebograhy on a patient, an accident was encountered during the procedure. While these procedures were performed under fluoroscopy on a tilt table, there was a malfunction and the table immobilized in the tilted erect position while the fluoroscopy was active. While the room was dark, my technician ran to the control panel. Both me and my assistant resident were in a panic and could hear our own breathing during that utter silence. All we could do to prevent the patient from falling was to hold the patient in erect posture. The only visible object was the lit screen with the image. The injected contrast visible on fluoroscopy was washed away by the inflowing blood, and that which was caught in the webs of the venous valves was clearly visible.

This attracted my attention, and to my dismay, noticed a rhythmic opening and closing of these valves occurring almost like the heart beat. I was overcome by this observation, which I in turn shared with my resident, as it was just a passing observation at that nervous moment. By the time the technician returned, everything fell into place, and we all took a sigh of relief. However, it was this passing observation, made during a nervous moment, which continued to haunt me, as it had no logical explanation.

I tried to reason if this motion is primary by the valves or secondary to some other external force. A fortnight later, it is like someone woke me up in the middle of the night saying, "look, there must be more to it, it is occurring rythmically like the cardiac cycle secondary to the heart." It is then, when I began to contemplate this phenomenon and began researching the history of venous valves. It was an amazing experience for me to realize that so much has been thought and written about venous valves and at various times and under various names, beginning with the time of Hippocrates. I will provide more detail written on this subject in a later chapter.

Exactly 400 hundred years earlier, the function of the venous valves was discovered by Fabricius Aquapendente. I was also curious to note the motion of the venous valves is hitherto unnoticed and unknown in the field of medicine. From this point forward, I started observing each patient undergoing descending phlebography and recording the motion in cine video, with the motion of the venous valves occurring during each rhythmic heartbeat. In some patients, the motion was subtle and in others very obvious, I could time the function of the venous valves with the patient's electrocardiogram and observed the opening of valves coinciding with the "P" waves. These valves opened during diastole and closed during systole of the atrium. I was not able to explain the reason for this motion, but, was very much convinced that it was not a primary motion but that of a secondary motion related to the function of the atrium. Years later I recorded the same motion in the popliteal valves by grey scale duplex scanning.

These findings motivated me to study the history of venous valves and conduct experiments on the canine heart to study the role of the atrial diastole on the circulation of blood in the venous system. I shall enumerate each of my new findings one by one in this treatise and share these experiments and their findings which lead me to this discovery.

For the next ten years, I was stifled, as I could not find a proper explanation to describe these new findings. There was no way, unless I visualized the assignment of the atrial chambers under an absolutely new dimension. A new understanding on the laws of muscle function, at least in the cardiac muscle fibers of atrium, was inevitable. My mind, like that of everybody's, was programmed in medical school by the great minds of the past who were considered the "Fathers of Modern Medicine." They laid down certain fundamental concepts well-ingrained in our brains and inerasable at the time. When I read the history, the time they spent and the struggle they faced to emerge from their traditional teaching, was the only inspiring force.

The famous experiment of Starling, wherein the electrical stimulation of the thigh muscle of the frog, causing a sudden contraction recording an upward graphic curve, is the basis of his theory that muscles contract and recoil back to their normal position in the resting phase, is the one experiment which is repeated by almost all students across the world in the physiology laboratory, and the concept that muscles only contract is ingrained in our brains. It took me a very long time to leap out of this box and realize, ultimately that muscles not only contract but also stretch, and both are active phenomena associated with the physiological, chemical and electrical changes at the cellular level. A key factor for me, was to assign a new function to the atrial diastole as an equally active phenomena of the cardiac cycle with a specific function.

Sir William Harvey focused his attention to the ventricular chambers in an attempt to unravel its function. The other two chambers of the heart, the atria, were established to be nonfunctional except that they performed as storage of blood for the ventricles. Historically, there is a valid reason for this; from the time of Aristotle, the anatomy of the human heart was described solely by the observation of the naked eye, and it was reported that there was a diametrical difference in the texture of the ventricles comparing to the structures of Atria adjacent to them. Further reports described the atrial wall, felt and resembled more like the vena cava than that of hard muscular and fibrous feeling of the solid ventricular chambers of the heart. It was firmly believed and described that the ventricular chambers make up the heart and atrial chambers described as extended pouches of vena cava rather than part of the heart. This teaching continued until the time of Sir William Harvey. May be the strong reason why He concentrated only on the Ventricles and assigned function of the Heart only to those two chambers. This is very clear further when he explained the reason for the existence of Mitral and tricuspid valve and its function to prevent leaking of blood back into the great veins during ventricular systole rather than mentioning back into the atrial chambers.

Medical school curriculum at the time Sir William Harvey was in Padua included the teachings of Aristotle's philosophy and anatomy, and Galen's physiology. Obviously, Sir William Harvey, graduating within those teachings, assigned the function of the heart to ventricular chambers and considered the atria as passive chambers functioning as collecting pools of blood. The atrial diastole was considered simply as the resting phase of the atria. This teaching holds true even today in medical schools, as does the teaching that ventricles do the mechanical function of pushing the blood forward to the pulmonary and systemic arteries, and in essence, act in a manner as forward pushing pumps.

Sir William Harvey's mentor, Fabricius Hieronymus Aquapendente, discovered the function of the venous valves almost 400 years prior, as they are one-way doors which prevents retrograde flow of blood into the venous tree. Therefore, once the blood reaches the veins it can only flow towards the heart. Sterling's famous experiment on a frog's leg, which was duplicated by almost every medical student in the physiology lab worldwide, inculcated the idea that muscles function only by the contraction of its fibers, and in the resting phase it is in a stretched mode. In other words, the stretched mode is functionless.

As a result of the above teachings, my experimental findings lacked explanation and expression. It was not until I allowed my thinking to go outside this box, which took almost ten years of repeated thought experiments, contemplation, disappointing moments, and a desperate search to find words of expression, that I was able to explain the motion of blood in the venous system. It was during this time that I was able to associate the rest of my discoveries to each other. Each of these events were related to each other, originating by the diastole of the atrial chambers. It was only after this association was made that I was able to present these new concepts in various national and international meetings.

In the beginning, my reported findings were rejected by many peer reviewed journals. However, this never hindered my enthusiasm, because it was a totally new understanding and finding. Initially, I expected resistance in order for my peers to digest and accept my findings. In 2009, my findings were accepted and published by the International Journal of Angiology.

During this journey, I began to research the history of venous valves. I won't be charged with exaggeration if I say the history of the venous valves almost covers the entire history of western medicine from the time of Aristotle to present day. It is the single most important factor used as the justification of the technical aspects of phlebotomy used in the treatment of ailments, particularly as it relates to infectious and contagious causes, and continued several decades past the time of Sir William Harvey. Ultimately, medical fraternities accepted the new theories of circulation reported by Sir William Harvey, and ultimately, the teachings of the heart replaced the liver as the organ of circulation in the human body.

Following the life of Sir William Harvey, his understanding of the function of venous valves from his teacher Aquapendente, and his obsession with the function of the venous valves, provided him insight into the circulation of blood in the human body, along with his historic concepts of the mechanical function of ventricles which affirmed the motion of blood in single closed circuit. It is not a wonder that in his written monologue on the function of the heart, that there is only one diagram, depicting the sole function of the venous valves of the superficial veins of the forearm. He also explains how he used this knowledge in various simple experiments to derive his conclusions.

It was a moment of joy for me to know the function of the valves inspired Sir William Harvey to discover the ventricular function of the heart, and almost 400 years later, the discovery of the motion of the venous valves inspired me to establish the function of atrial diastole of the human heart; an intriguing historical connection of the discoveries. This will further complement and complete our knowledge on the mechanical function of the heart and open new doors in the world of research to a better understanding and treatment of ailments affecting the human heart.

chapter one

The history of circulation

I realized upon initiating an epistemological search of the history of circulation that it is essential for me to share with you the chronological events as they relate to the newly discovered findings of my experimental work and also give the history a proper perspective.

The founding concepts of circulation of the allopathic science of medicine originate in the doctrines conveyed by the giant personality of his time, the great Aristotle. That does not mean there was no comprehension of circulation prior to Aristotle but it is not relevant to the changes we seek following the new findings as reported in my work.

I am sure Aristotle himself looked over his shoulders at the teaching of his elders. His father was a physician to the king of Macedonia and therefore was exposed to the teachings of biology, physiology, and anatomy very early in his life. He later became a student of Plato.

Phases of the history of circulation

The history of circulation can be divided into three phases. The first phase spans from the time of Hippocrates to that of Galen. Several great minds of the time played an important role during the period 384 BC to 120 AD. In addition to Aristotle, many other noble and well-equipped minds were active in the study such as **Praxagoras** in 340 BC run in Herophillius and Erasistratus, both in the 3rd century BC, contributed to and improvised the findings of Aristotle. They performed cadaver dissections to confirm their findings. They mostly complemented the concepts conveyed by Aristotle or generated new ideas based on his theories.

The theory of circulation—pre-Galenic era

Aristotle's theory of medicine revolves around the doctrines of four basic qualities of the human body: hot, cold, wet, and dry. Homeostasis of these four qualities in a human body is the

DOI: 10.1201/b22792-1

cornerstone of health according to Aristotle. The basis of medical treatment was as a means to correct and balance these qualities in a diseased state. Later thinkers such as Galen believed in these four principles of the body and gave them different names such as the four humors and the four temperaments. The most important gift Aristotle gave to future generations of scientists was his affirmation of the superiority of facts over theory. He declared to his students that if there was a newly discovered fact that contradicted any past or even age-old theory then the theory must be modified or if need be discarded. This is a very encouraging statement and aided me to report on my discovery of these new experimental findings. These findings may contradict or complement the theories laid down by those great human minds who preceded me.

Aristotle, according to his observation in a chick embryo, established the heart as the first organ to be formed in the body. He described it as a three-chambered organ and as the center of vitality in the body. Somehow all these authors were convinced that the warmth of the body was generated by the heart, and when heart stops, the body cools down and the person dies. They hypothesized that the heart circulates pneuma (air) and vital spirit through the arteries to the rest of the body. They also postulated that the human body needs nourishment to live. This postulation was a great step forward since until that time it was thought that nourishment was derived from the divine causation rather than the absorption of food into the intestines. It was the first time ever described that nourishment is derived from the intestines and goes to the liver where blood is manufactured and the origin of veins from the liver carry nourishment and humor or temperaments to the rest of the body. Maintaining the balance of these four temperaments is the secret of good health. Originally, Aristotle named all vessels as veins. Later, Praxagoras was the first to name arteries and veins separately. The understanding of the time was that arteries begin in the heart and carry pneuma and vital spirit to the rest of the body, but they did not give credit to the flow of blood in the arteries. They considered the spirit of life as the vital force, and pneuma flowed in the arteries and was diffused to the tissues. They believed that the liver played the central role and blood flowed from there centrifugally with the vena cava ascending up from the liver and taking blood to the heart, brain, and lungs. Then the vena cava descending downward takes blood to the rest of the body tissues. The atrium was not considered to be a separate chamber and part of the heart. They believed the vena cava carried blood to the brain, heart, and lungs at the junction of the ventricles, which expanded to a pouch and served as a collection and delivery area of the blood to the ventricles. Hence the atria were described as an extension and part of the vena cava and pulmonary veins rather than a separate chamber of the heart. To further support their thinking, observation of the atrial wall with the naked eye resembled the vena cava rather than the ventricles with the exception of a small non-functioning appendage, which they named the auricle as it appeared to be an extension and remnant of the ventricle. Therefore, all explanations and teachings of the heart were based on two ventricles. This teaching influenced Sir William Harvey as well and was grounded in a genuine reason. The syllabus of the medical school in Padua consisted of subjects of anatomy, philosophy, and physiology written by Aristotle and Galen. Harvey fostered those teachings and his experiments of the heart were mainly concentrated on the ventricles.

The above teaching about the atrium continues to the present time and the atrium was never given a functional importance. Modern anatomists definitely described the atria as two separate chambers of the heart and not as an extension of the vena cava. That is the only progress that has been made at the anatomical level. At present, the heart is described as a four-chambered organ.

The anatomical structure of the heart was defined by Aristotle and the rest of the stalwarts who followed him continued his teachings. Aristotle defined the heart as hard flesh not easily injured and composed of hard and tense muscular fibers. That definition surpassed all the others. Definitely only two chambers of the heart, the right and left ventricles, corresponded to that description of the heart with the exception of the auricle of the atrium, which appears to be an appendage of the ventricle. The remainder of the atrium did not even come close to it and was never considered to be a functional part of the heart. Sir William Harvey did not devote any importance to the atrial chambers in his theory of the explanation of the motion of blood in the body. He concentrated his efforts solely on the ventricular chambers. He thought of the atria as a storage house for blood. Up to the end of Galen's era, all anatomists believed that the arteries and veins were end vessels and diffused into the tissues.

Vital spirits flowing to the end arteries are continuously dissipated into the tissues. We can generalize the theory of the circulation during the pre-Galenic era as explained in the diagram (Figure 1.1). Nourishment is taken from the intestine via the portal vein to the liver and it transforms this nourishment into blood and distributes it to various parts of the body through the hepatic vein and into the vena cava. The ascending portion of the vena cava supplies the heart, brain, and lungs. The descending portion of the vena cava supplies the rest of the body. The left ventricle and arteries are thought to be devoid of blood. It distributes the pneuma and life spirit to the rest of the body. Both the arteries and veins are thought to be end vessels and diffuse into the tissues. These were the concepts and teachings of circulation at the time. Based upon this, various ailments were treated (Figure 1.1).

The theory of circulation—Galenic era

Bloodletting was practiced early on to eliminate the excess of humor in the blood and to establish equilibrium as a method of treatment to restore the health of a patient. This continued until the 2nd century AD, at which time there came a great mind in the history of medicine, a child prodigy, Claudius Galen was born in 129 AD in Pergamum, Asia Minor (presently Bergama, western Turkey) during the peak of the Roman Empire. At the age of 16 he became a medical student. He traveled abroad seeking knowledge, and his studies brought him to the famous School of Medicine in Alexandria, Egypt. Galen returned home and held the prestigious post of surgeon to the Gladiators. His ambitions took him on a quest to become a celebrity seeking fame and fortune. Galen was a voracious writer and covered subjects ranging from medicine, through logic, philosophy, and literature. He gave public demonstrations on the art of medicine. These activities catapulted him to such fame that he was appointed Physician of the Emperor.

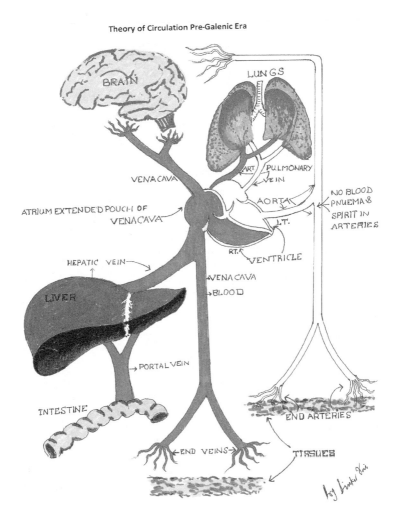

Figure 1.1 Theory of circulation in the pre-Galenic era. Nourishment is taken from the intestine via the portal vein. The liver transforms this nourishment into blood and distributes it to various parts of the body through the hepatic vein.

Galen established his own doctrines on the subjects he taught. He mainly conducted dissections on apes and pigs. He revived the teachings and methods of treatment established by all the past Greek physicians and philosophers from the time of

Hippocrates onward. His authority and influence were such that his theories of circulation lived unchallenged and unquestioned almost 1,300 years, at which time Sir William Harvey entered the scene.

Galen modified most of the old doctrines and gave a specific name and form to them and explained them in his own and very candid method. He demonstrated that the body is made of four definite humors which were not addressed until then, although the same concept since the time of Hippocrates had been practiced under various presumptions. Galen named them black bile, yellow bile, blood, and phlegm. A proper balance of these four humors in the human body is the hallmark of good health according to him. Based on that, he discussed "theory of Plenitude and Plethora." During his time bloodletting as the main method of balancing of these humors became a very well-practiced treatment of many ailments and especially in the management of contagious diseases. He described various techniques of phlebotomy to various parts of the body to suit different ailments. He was the first to accept, in addition to pneuma and vital spirits that there is also blood in the arteries. He could not discard blood's obvious presence in the arteries and therefore he postulated a theory to describe the presence of blood in the left ventricle. The interventricular septum has pores through which some blood passes from the right ventricle to the left ventricle and flows to the arteries. However he did not give credit to it as the main content of the arteries. Galen still thought the pneuma comes from the lungs and the vital spirit from the heart. He might have derived this concept from his observation of the foramen oval in the mammalian fetal heart and might have thought that it continues to stay as invisible pores in the interventricular septum during the growth of the fetus.

It was Realdo Colombo (1516–1559), an Italian professor of anatomy and surgeon at the University of Padua, Rome, Italy, who established the pulmonary circulation, modulated by describing how venous blood of the right ventricle passes through the lung and reaches the left ventricle. According to Galen, the heart was the cauldron of the body. The heart warmed the blood and as it got warmer it ebbed out of the cauldron and overflowed into the vessels, like milk when boiled ebbs and flows out of the kettle, and was thus famously known as the ebb and flow theory of Galen (Figure 1.2). So Galen did not attribute any mechanical

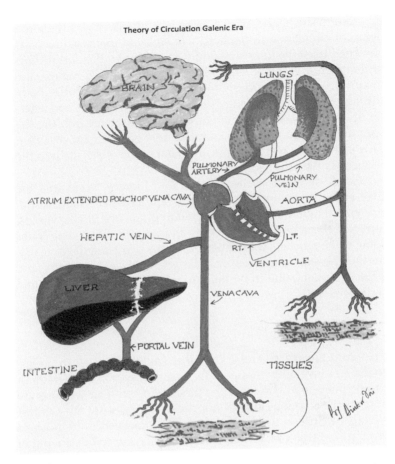

Figure 1.2 Theory of circulation Galenic era. According to Galen, the heart is the hot pot. Arterial blood derived from the right ventricle warms up and webs out to the arteries and flows into the tissues and carries pneuma and vital spirits by diffusing them to the tissues in the arteries. A portion is distributed to the lungs and the brain carrying the psychic spirit, with the remaining amount going to all the other organs and tissues of the body. The liver is the main organ of circulation and continuously manufactures blood containing nutrition and the additional four humors; blood, black bile, yellow bile, and phlegm, which matches Aristotle's concept of the four temperaments. Galen called this the "animal spirit." Blood flows from the vena cava and is carried with all its components to the heart, lungs, brain, and other organs and tissues of the body. Blood is diffused to the tissues through these end vessels and is continuously reproduced and replaced as needed.

function to the heart. According to him, the liver was the main organ of circulation in the body. He believed that nutrition was absorbed from the intestines and was carried by the portal veins to the liver. It is in the liver where blood and other humors are manufactured continuously and distributed to the entire body through the veins. According to Galen both the veins and arteries are end vessels, and therefore blood dissipates into the tissues and is continuously produced and replaced by the liver. This is the same way pneuma and vital spirits dissipate into the tissues via the arteries.

Galen declared to the medical and literary world that the liver is the organ supporting circulation and the Arabic world, primarily embodied by the Persian, Egyptian, and Arabic worlds, attracted the attention of the poets and writers of that time. Later some of these beliefs were inherited by the Urdu language created by the "Mogul" emperors of India who were of Persian origin. That is how it came to be known among the Indian poets and writers as well.

Historical impact

The word "liver" in Arabic *(kabed)* is frequently used in poetry to express love and emotional feeling. A common expression of lovers, poets, and writers of the time, the word liver was used to express the emotions of love. A lover saying "you are my KALEJA (liver)" in Urdu is used extensively and practiced even today in poetry. An Arabic expression of a father saying to his son out of love goes like this: *"Baba cal lewalado anta falzat KEBED (liver)."* The English translation is "you are my part of my liver, son." All these various expressions were derived from the unknown influence of Galen. Such sayings are equivalent to today's expression, *"you are the love in my heart"* which is derived from the work of Harvey, who declared that the heart is the main organ of circulation. This is so much so that today love is symbolized as a human heart. This is a very interesting historical interconnection of events which I noticed and wove into my quest for the evolution of the theories of circulation.

According to the teachings of Galen, blood flowed away centrifugally in the veins to various parts of the body and was diffused into the tissues and never returned. The arteries and veins are thought to be end vessels and separate circulatory systems. An imbalance in the humors and the flow of blood was thought to be the main cause of many ailments, specifically the contagious and infectious components. Bloodletting was the common treatment of the time. A circulatory system powered by a pumping mechanism of the heart was never contemplated. During the next 1,500 years these theories and concepts went unchallenged and were upheld even after the deaths of Galen as well as that of Sir William Harvey. It is intriguing to me how generation after generation almost for the next 1,500 years were the blind followers of this system. Going through the historical events of first 1500 AC we can put out various theories that played a role that is not relevant and is a separate subject.

But suffice it to say here that this is a learning point that communicates that scientific reasoning is fragile and can be suppressed under political, theological, and cultural conditions. He died at the age of 80 in 210 AD. His studies were confined to that of living or dead animals. In keeping with the tradition of Aristotle's teachings, Galen believed in deductive logic to arrive at many conclusions. Sometimes his premise was wrong, hence this spread to his conclusions. The most evident of them is his theory of the heart, that is that it is the hottest organ in the body and warmth dissipates from the heart to the rest of the body. This deduction might have been correct if the heart were really the hottest organ in the body but it is not, yet surprisingly this went unchallenged for 1,500 years. One can only speculate perhaps that there were no specific tools to monitor the temperature of the body or to confirm the temperature of the entire human body. Galen coined the heart *"a hot cauldron—blood warming pot."* Warm blood ebbed and overflowed into the arteries, with blood overflowing rather than circulating in a closed system. Through the arteries the blood delivered pneuma collected from the lungs and vital spirit that originated from the heart.

As a matter of fact, in order for a physician to carry out the treatment of various types of venesection to various parts of the body, it is fundamentally dependent upon the ebb and flow theory of Galen. Consequently, this theory was never questioned even after Sir William Harvey's revolutionary discoveries. According to Harvey air egressed through the pulmonary veins to the left ventricle because the left atria considered to be the end portion of the pulmonary vein. Similarly, the right atrium is a part of the vena cava and its role is to store and drain blood into the right ventricle. At the same time vapors regressed to the lungs, carrying vital spirits from the left ventricle. The animal spirits manufactured in the liver were distributed to all organs and tissues of the body by the veins. This was the concept of circulation during the Galenic era.

chapter two

Sir William Harvey

Background

William Harvey was a brilliant Englishman born on April 1, 1578, in Folkestone, Kent, England, at the beginning of the Renaissance Period. He followed a new path that laid the foundation of modern medicine and opened new doors that required experimental evidence that were imperative for establishing a scientific foundation. Harvey followed his analysis with hypotheses that were supported by direct repetitive experimental evidence. He matriculated as a student at Gonville and Caius College, Cambridge, where he studied the arts and medicine. After receiving his Bachelor of Arts degree in 1599, he traveled to Italy to study medicine at the University of Padua, the leading European medical school at the time. The curriculum of the medical school included Galen's philosophy and physiology and Aristotle's anatomy. Harvey became a student of the Italian anatomist and surgeon, Hieronymous Fabricius Acquapendente. He had considerable influence on Harvey.

Acquapendente was the first to discover the function of the venous valves in the superficial veins of the foot.[1] He described them as "one-way doors allowing blood to flow in one direction, toward the heart, and preventing regress." This discovery bestowed on Fabricius a celebrity status and helped to his appointment to the Chair of the University. Fabricius' discovery appears likely to have played a major role in Harvey's future work on the theory of the circulation of blood. It is likely that he was exposed to the demonstration of the function of the venous valves even before their discovery was published in 1603 by his teacher. During the same time that Harvey was at the University of Padua, Galileo was the Chairman of the Department of Mathematics. Since he was fascinated with valvular function, Harvey used it in his many experiments to establish his theories of circulation. In his entire book there is only one diagram, that which depicts

DOI: 10.1201/b22792-2

the venous valves in superficial veins of the forearm. There is no doubt Harvey learned the method of exhibiting the motion of blood in veins flowing in one direction toward the heart by a simple strip test from Fabricius and will be explained later in the various experiments he conducted.

Methods

A soft tourniquet is applied above the elbow to occlude the superficial vein, thereby distending the distal veins of the forearm. In doing so the sites of valves were clearly exhibited as small intermittent bulges along the course of each vein. One can pick one of the veins and distally occlude it with finger pressure. Gently using the other finger of the free hand, one squeezes the vein proximally beyond one of the valves by running it upward toward the tourniquet; this releases pressure. The collapsed vein begins to fill retrograde but only up to the most proximal valve, and the segment below remains collapsed. This demonstrated how the valves prevent regress of blood. Upon releasing the proximal finger pressure one can notice how the collapsed distal segment of the vein fills once again, revealing venous blood flows from the distal part of the vein proximally toward the heart. This is called a "STRIP TEST" which is utilized to check the competency of the venous valves in vein valve transplant surgery. This experiment leads to the famous discovery by Fabricius on the function of venous valves in the venous tree. In the diagram (Figure 2.1), Harvey utilized the same tourniquet tests, modifying them to prove his theories with experimental evidence. The teachings of Aristotle and Galen continued to influence Harvey and most likely played a role in overlooking certain areas. Harvey was able to discard some of Hippocrates', Aristotle's, and later Galen's doctrines of circulation utilizing his experiments with several tourniquet tests, and the knowledge of which in principle he inherited from his mentor Fabricius.

The following doctrines of Galen and the ancient Greeks remained uncontested until such time. Their teachings were:

1. Veins contain blood produced in the liver and arteries contain vital spirits and pneuma.
2. According to Galen, the right ventricle is designed for a private function to provide blood to the lungs for nutrition. In

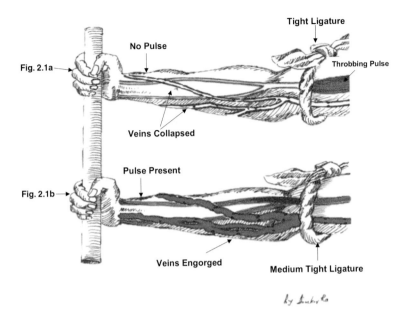

Figure 2.1 Schematic of Harvey's experiments with ligatures. Harvey employed tight ligatures (top Figure 2.1a) to totally occlude the arteries and veins in the arm leading to the hand. This resulted in reduced blood flow distally and no radial and ulnar pulses. In addition, all veins proximal and distal to the ligature collapsed. The hand became pale and cold. The artery proximal to the ligature is shown throbbing. He employed medium tight ligatures (bottom Figure 2.1b) to occlude only the veins, resulting in unimpaired arterial flow of blood to the extremities but impairing venous drainage. The arterial pulse at the wrist is intact, while the distal veins are seen as distended. The hand becomes swollen and deeply colored.

contrast, the left ventricle is designed to supply vital spirits. Unlike the ancient Greeks, Galen accepted the presence of blood in the arteries as an addition rather than as the main content. He postulated that blood came from the right to the left ventricle through invisible pores in the interventricular septum which divided them.

3. All the scientists of this period were convinced that there was no connection between arteries and veins as they were end vessels, both merging into the tissues with blood permeating the tissues for nourishment.

4. The liver continuously manufactured blood.
5. No one appreciated the mechanical nature of the heart.
6. Galen popularized the ebb and flow theory of circulation. This provided the basis for venesection as a treatment of diseases by bloodletting.

Experimental revelation of Sir William Harvey

We can time and time again marvel at the genius of Harvey and his courage to discard one-by-one the age-old theories of his masters whom he continued to hold in high reverence. His experimental evidence and the teachings of Fabricius aided him to reach his conclusions.[2]

Harvey applied two types of ligatures (tourniquets) on the arm (Figure 2.1).[3]

The first was a tight ligature which occluded both veins and arteries, resulting in a loss of a distal pulse of the arteries. He observed the distal limb which became pale, and that the distal veins had collapsed. In the second test he applied a softer ligature of medium tightness, and just tight enough to occlude only the veins. An arterial pulse was still palpable distally and the distal veins were immediately distended. With these two tests aided by the naked eye observation, he concluded that blood enters the arm by the arteries and leaves by the veins. Harvey affirmed for the first time that there is communication between the arteries and veins through minute porosities in the tissues without loss of blood.

Harvey was the first to discover anastomosis between arteries and veins with the above simple experiment even before the discovery of capillaries. At the time, his discovery was met with much skepticism. He never succeeded in tracing any connection between the arteries and veins by direct anastomoses because the table microscope later used to evaluate tissues had not yet been developed. The controversy surrounding Harvey's model for the circulation of blood persisted until Marcello Malpighi's discovery of capillaries in 1661 in the lungs.

The medical world helplessly had to accept the genius and uncanny foresight of Sir William Harvey. It was not easy for Harvey to stand up against the most popular and well-accepted teachings of his predecessors. It took a while for him to interpret his new discoveries and assign a form and new descriptive light to them.

Anticipating opposition to his revolutionary theories, Harvey wrote in his book *"Not only do I fear danger to myself from malice of a few, but I dread lest I have fallen all men as enemies."*

The next great discovery

The next great discovery involved the ventricular function of the heart. Harvey focused solely on ventricular function because he was still under the influence of Aristotle's anatomy of the heart, which he had learned as a student at Padua. Those who followed Aristotle's anatomical description of the heart believed that it was made of two ventricular chambers and that the atria are an extension of the vena cava on the right side and the pulmonary vein on the left side. The atrial wall structure is thin and the ventricular wall structure is fibrous, thick, hard, and strong. They did not resemble each other sufficiently for Aristotle to incorporate them as one organ. Harvey observed during ventricular systole that the heart becomes erect, can rise upward, and strikes at the chest when contracted. When felt between the fingers, it becomes hard. During contraction, the left ventricle flushes blood into the aorta to flow to the rest of the body. Similarly, the right ventricle flushes blood into the pulmonary artery to reach the lungs. This expulsion of blood with force expands the arterial system of the body, which he termed arterial diastole. He discarded the past theories of dual circulation and instead made the most monumental discovery that the circulation of blood takes place in a closed circuit—starting at the left ventricular systole and running through the arteries, flowing in the veins, and then back to the right ventricle. Harvey, by measuring the volume of the ventricle, was able to approximately estimate the volume of blood flowing through and being expelled during each systole. He then estimated an ejection fraction giving credit to minimal to maximal possibilities and then concluded that the amount of blood that circulates through the heart is enormously more in both possibilities and more than the actual volume present in the body. This further ascertained his conviction that the heart is a closed circulatory system and contains a given volume of blood present in the body that keeps circulating continuously without any loss in the tissues. This was a major breakthrough from the past.

As far as the anatomy of the heart is concerned, Harvey remained under the influence of his past teachers, Aristotle and Galen, who believed that the heart is made up of two ventricles. As described today, the atria were thought to be the extension of the vena cava on the right side and the venous arteria venosa (pulmonary vein) on the left side. The texture of the wall of the atria resembled the wall of the vena cava with the exception of a small portion known as the auricles or ears. The auricles were functionless and were fibrous and thick like the ventricle. Therefore even Harvey did not give any functional importance to the atrial chambers. The atria they addressed are the auricular part that we anatomically include today as part of the atrial chambers and consider as the remnants of ventricle. The function or role of the atria was never discussed by Harvey, nor did he declare that the atria are functionless. He continued to accept that it is the extended portion of the vena cava and collects blood before it goes into the ventricles, as is well explained in his book. Generations later, anatomists clearly defined the heart as an organ with four chambers. They also continued to describe the atria as the collecting chambers and the auricles as the remnants to fit into the doctrines of Harvey, who had established the function of the ventricle. The ventricles are the functioning chambers and forward pushing pumps, giving the legacy to Harvey. Harvey did credit the ventricle for the circulation of blood in the entire circuit composed of arteries and veins. He was also thoroughly convinced that the ventricular contraction expelled blood with such force that it circulated in the closed system back to the right ventricle after circling through the arteries and veins. Harvey convinced himself that nature created venous valves within the veins serving as a function of "one-way doors" preventing the regress of blood. He thought that ultimately the blood has to reach the atrium with a single forward pushing force of ventricular systole.

Intermittent systolic contraction of the ventricles creates pulsation along the arteries and slows down in the veins as the force of expulsion is diminished at the end of the circuit. Harvey thought that the forward pushing force of the ventricles was adequate to keep the blood in motion within the arteries and veins and return it to the atria. This theory was given credence for a long time. Later, researchers measuring the force of the ventricles realized that the contraction force of the ventricles disappeared by the time blood reached the veins through the capillaries. This was more evident when the blood in the veins would have to overcome gravitational force. Ventricular contraction, even at its peak, would dissipate by the time blood reached the venous part of the circuit. If ventricular contraction was the only force, the weight of the blood in the veins would overcome the ventricular forward pushing force and blood would remain stagnant in the veins. Harvey's theories were well established and as a result the forces contributing to the motion of blood in the veins against the force of gravity remained a mystery for a long time.

Sir William Harvey dispelled age-old theories of circulation held by Aristotle and his generation and then by Galen and the generations to follow. For more than 1,300 years Galen's views dominated medical opinion and entire generations of physicians did not question obedient students of his teaching. Harvey's work was the model of accurate observation, careful experimentation, and notation with logical interpretation. He had a passion for anatomy and believed that full knowledge of it would open the doors to the secrets of circulation.

Acquapendente became a celebrity and famous anatomist after his discovery of the function of the venous valves. This discovery catapulted him into the position of the Chair of the Department of Anatomy at Padua University. At the time Harvey traveled from England in search of higher learning. The discovery of valvular function by his teacher played an important role in his discovery of ventricular function of the heart. Harvey learned the art of dissection from Fabricius, who was the great master of the art. Harvey devoted his time to a meticulous and continuous series of dissections, mainly concentrating on the circulatory systems of a wide variety of animals. He amassed an enormous amount of information on the comparative anatomy of the heart and blood vessels which was thus far unknown for the rest of his time or for the researchers who preceded him. His interpretation and new discoveries stunned the medical and scientific communities. It drove the physicians of his time to the brink of collapse and to practice medical science based on the theories of Galen. It led to such a conspiracy among physicians that Harvey, on the eve of his disclosure of the mechanical function of the heart and motion of the blood in the human body learned of his planned assassination by the Royal Court. Hence Harvey had to flee overnight from the United Kingdom to France.

During the next two years, Harvey lived anonymously. It was during this time that he decided to record his work for posterity and in the form of a monologue. He wrote in Latin, a short book titled *De Mortu Cordis and De Circulatione Sanguinis*.[4] Harvey published the book in 1628 in Frankfurt, Germany. He subsequently wrote two more volumes under the phrase of exercitations twenty years later in 1649 entitled *De Circulatione Sanguinis*. He referred them to John Riolan primarily as a rebuttal to his critics. Harvey's monologue is honored as one of the one hundred great books of Western civilization. During his time, the only scientific discoveries granted recognition and authenticity were those accepted for presentation at the Royal Court in the presence of the King. Although it surprised the contemporary medical world, it did not change the practice of medicine based on his theories.

Galen's teaching and practice of medicine continued long after Harvey's death. Slowly over the years his practices influenced the wisdom of future generations of physicians. At the beginning of the 18th century, it was considered that anything that had been written and/or practiced prior to Harvey was worthy of consideration. The great Dutch teacher of medicine in Leiden, Herman Boerhaave, stated that before Harvey both Aristotle and Galen addressed arteries as veins. Harvey named arteries as an arterial vein and veins as a vein. All contractions of the heart were named systole and dilatation as diastole. Diastole was also used to describe arterial vein pulsation. Harvey focused mainly on the ventricular systole since all his findings were based upon naked eye observations. He could only concentrate on one aspect of the heart during his observations. Harvey is also quoted as saying, "it is not humanly possible to observe the motion of all the chambers of the heart simultaneously. So henceforth, I shall concentrate only on the motion of ventricles." As far as the atrium was concerned, Harvey was very much influenced by the anatomical descriptions taught by Aristotle and Galen: the atria were an extension of the vena cava draining blood directly into the ventricles. Harvey did not consider the mechanical function of the atrium, if any. He had also not discussed any functional role of the atria.

Harvey made his first and the most important observation; when ventricles contract the arterial vein arising both from the right and left ventricles they dilate simultaneously; he called this diastole. During his experiment, when an artery was cut, blood spurted out with increased force like a fountain. This experiment led him to conclude that ventricular systole thrusts blood forward and this is the main and the only force that keeps blood in motion in the body within the close circuit created by the arteries and veins. He used the function of the venous valves to support his theory. This led Harvey to make a historical statement to his contemporary chemist and friend, Robert Boyle: "But for the understanding of the function of the venous valves, I would not have been able to prove my theory." Perhaps this is the reason he devotes his utmost importance to the venous valves, and in his entire book there is only one diagram that is dedicated to the demonstration of the function of the venous valves and the adaptation of a series of tourniquet tests to conclude his theories of circulation. Harvey had not conducted any further anatomical dissections on the specimens of the heart or vessels, nor are there any further diagrams. By experimenting with dissections on various animals, he had established that blood leaves the heart and travels along the closed circuit formed by the arteries and veins. He found that the vessels that take blood from the ventricles are arterial veins, and the vessels that bring it back to the heart are veins. Through a series of dissections on various animals and dead bodies, he declared that both arteries and veins are connected and blood flows out from the left ventricle and returns to the right ventricle through the closed channels. This convinced Harvey that the ventricular force ultimately pushes blood back into the heart and the valves were created to serve the purpose of preventing blood from regressing (Figure 2.2).

Theory of circulation by Sir William Harvey

The medical world following the teachings of Harvey taught that the ventricles were the only two chambers that conduct the mechanical function of the forward pushing motion and the heart was the forward pushing pump of the body. After Harvey, this was the first time a mechanical organ was identified in the human body. Future anatomists are credited with the establishment of

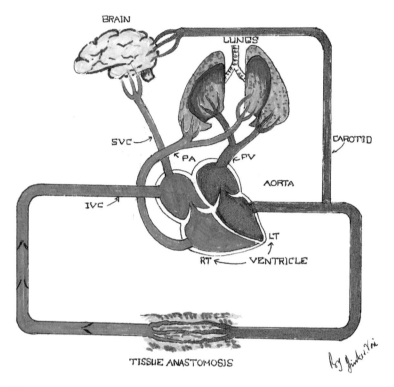

Figure 2.2 Theory of circulation by Sir William Harvey. PA=pulmonary artery; PV=pulmonary vein; SVC=superior vena cava; IVC=inferior vena cava. Arteries and veins anastomose in the tissues and form a closed circulatory system. The left ventricular systole is the sole force of circulation of blood in the systemic arterial venous system. The right ventricular systole is the force of circulation of blood in the pulmonary system.

the theory that the human heart consists of four chambers: two atria and two ventricles. The auricles or "ears" in Latin are remnants of the ventricle that were previously described as part of the atrial chambers.

To feature the functional description of Harvey, even at the present time the atrial chambers were considered passive chambers storing blood and that the atrial diastole is the resting phase. Blood flows from the vena cava and pulmonary veins and is stored first in these chambers before flowing to the corresponding ventricles. Harvey's conclusions were made from open dissections of the heart of mostly mammals, fish, and serpents. He depended upon his findings by observations of the naked eye. There were no experimental models, monitors, or table microscopes of any kind during his time. Future generations to come marveled of the genius of Sir William Harvey and his work and discoveries, which gained even greater veneration. He was able to capture the function of ventricular contractions by doing experiments and observing the ejection of blood under pressure. He rightly established the forward pushing pump mechanism of ventricular systole which has stood the test of time. He did not notice any other force that shared in the process of circulation. Harvey's conclusion was that ventricular contraction is the one underlying cause for the motion of blood and its circulation in arteries.

chapter three

Present concept

Physiologists who followed the time of Harvey realized that the ventricular force exerted in systole is good enough to take blood to the terminal arterioles into the capillaries and then vanish. If ventricular force was the sole force of circulation, the weight of the venous column of blood would neutralize and stagnation of blood in the venous system would occur. There would be no further motion of blood in the venous system (Figure 3.1).

Over the years, the medical world tried to attribute other forces to be responsible for the motion of blood in the venous tree. They realized that muscular contraction increases the velocity of venous blood by contracting the venous plexus embedded in the muscles, thereby contributing to an adjunctive force. The muscles of the calf became very prominent contributors since the popliteal and gastrocnemius muscles constantly contract while walking. A large volume of venous plexus is embedded in these muscles.

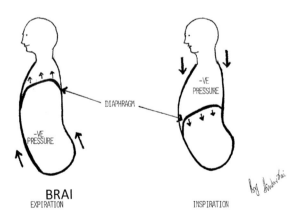

Figure 3.1 Upward and downward movement of the diaphragm creating alternating negative pressures in the abdomen and chest. This is responsible for venous return rather than respiration.

DOI: 10.1201/b22792-3

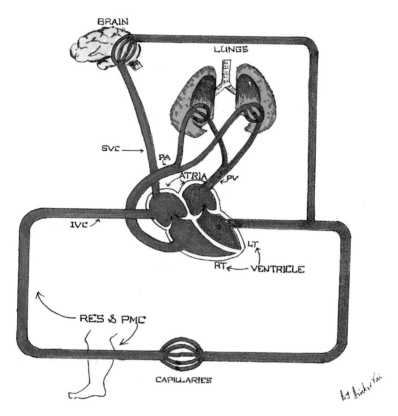

Figure 3.2 The theory of circulation at present. PA = pulmonary artery; PV = vein; SVC = superior vena cava; IVC = inferior vena cava; RES & pmc = respiration and peripheral muscular contraction (pump). These are the main forces of systemic venous circulation. The forces behind pulmonary venous return are unexplained. Both atria are blood collecting chambers and have no mechanical function. Ventricular systolic force pushes the blood forward into the arteries. This force is exhausted by the time it reaches the capillaries. Blood is thought to move in the veins back into the atrium by respiration and peripheral muscular contraction. At present the atrium is considered only a passive receptacle, and the heart is just a forward pushing pump.

Thus it was accepted as the main factor of venous circulation and it became popularly known as the "PERIPHERAL HEART OF THE BODY." This remained an unsatisfactory explanation, and researchers continued to search for other forces in an attempt to explain the motion of blood in the veins while in the resting state. Bollinger et al. in 1970[24] observed another important force aiding in the venous return of blood to the right atrium. He named it the abdominal thoracic two-phase pump.

During expiration the diaphragm moves up, decreasing intra-abdominal pressure, and the blood from the femoral veins of the lower extremities moves into the inferior vena cava. During inspiration the intrathoracic pressure further decreases and blood from the upper extremities moves into the superior vena cava (Figure 3.2). Since the work of Sir William Harvey over the last 400 years, there have been only two adjunctive forces identified and added to the explanation of the motion of blood in the venous tree. This leaves the door open as to the explanation of the main force responsible for keeping the blood in motion. The cause of venous return to the atrium remained a mystery.

chapter four

Mystery of the venous valves

My discovery of the motion of the venous valves that was observed as a passing phenomenon while performing a descending phlebography on a patient aroused a deep curiosity in my mind. Ultimately it was this observation that provided me with the first clue of the role of the atrium in the venous circulation. This observation constantly haunted me and ultimately it felt necessary for me to pursue the cause of motion of the venous valves. This was followed by a long gap. It was during this period that I developed an experimental model on mongrel canines and continued the dissection of canines, conducting a series of experiments that are described in detail in this section and in subsequent chapters.

In preliminary experiments, collecting and recording data was a tedious task. However, it was less of an ordeal compared to what I had to go through to interpret and solve the puzzle within the scope of the established concepts of the circulation of blood and the laws of muscle contraction established by well-developed minds of the past. During our training in medical school we considered these writers as sages of the past and placed them on the highest pedestal of teaching. Our entire thinking grew from within the premises of those established doctrines of the past. It took quite some time of contemplation and mental arguments before I could ultimately jump out of that box and rationalize these new findings and put them in order and into proper perspective. I tried to seek clarity and support from every possible source.

During one of those efforts I attempted to go through the history of venous valves in detail, which provided the most enlightening information. I was bewildered to find that it played a similar role in the experiments and the pursuits of William Harvey, leading him to discover the mechanical function of the ventricular systole of the heart. I was dismayed to read his letter to his friend, the famous chemist Robert Boyle, in which he

DOI: 10.1201/b22792-4

states, "But for the understanding of the function of the venous valves I would not have been able to prove my theory." Accepting his own words that the discovery he made on ventricular contraction and the laws of circulation of blood in arteries and veins was primarily dependent on his understanding of the function of the venous valves. This inspired me to pursue the new finding of motion of venous valves. When one peruses the history of medicine there is no subject both more contentious and contributory than the discovery of venous valves. When one searches throughout the history it is baffling to find that the entire progress as it relates to the area of circulation took place during the 16th and 17th centuries and revolves primarily around the subject of the venous valves. However insignificant venous valves appear in the human body, the discoveries made that gave way to our knowledge of the circulatory system were inspired by this one subject more than any other. It is this discovery that is all the more enigmatic. Without knowing the past history, almost 400 years later I stumbled on a similar experience in 1986 following the discovery of the motion of venous valves while conducting a descending phlebography in a patient. However casual an observation it was at the time it later inspired me to conduct a series of experiments in canines to trace the forces behind it. These experiments opened up a new discovery on the atrial diastolic function of the human heart and contributed new concepts to the motion of blood in the venous system and the laws of muscle contraction of the heart.

Ever since the practice of venous bloodletting arose as a method of treatment at the time of Hippocrates (460–370 BC),[5] the mention of the venous valves was made under different names and at different times. Assigning a function to the valves was the single most important factor involved in the controversial practice of venesection as a primary method of the treatment in the cure of some diseases for which Galen provided the indications and Antyllus provided the operative procedures.[6] Hence this became the most prominent method of treatment during Galen's era of the discovery of the function of venous valves since little doors preventing the regress of blood in veins weakened the ebb and flow theory of Galen on circulation. This was the important basis for phlebotomy as the main treatment for many infectious and contagious illnesses and one of the most important of Galen's time and studies and the widespread practice of physicians of the time all over Europe. Venous valves were initially called *Venorum Ostioles* and thought to be the thickening of the walls in veins. At the time it was not given any importance as to their function except for their ability to strengthen the walls of the veins. As long as Galen's theories dominated the scene of medicine for nearly 1,500 years that would contradict his diathesis known as *"Plethora and Plenitude,"* for which venesection was practiced based on the "ebb and flow" theory of the circulation of blood.

Cailiuse Orleans informs us that Erasistratus from the School of Chios (310–250 BC) discovered the existence of venous valves. Then later he led his students to discard the practice of venesection.[7] Charles Estienne (1503–1564 AC), descendent of a great scholarly French family, for the first time made a clear mention of the existence of venous valves in his work *De Dissectione Partium Corporis Humani.*[8] Since then, it became an important subject of research and the writing of many celebrated professors who chaired anatomy and surgery departments of the prestigious universities of Padua, Ferrara, Rome, and elsewhere. The dispute was not centered around their existence in the hepatic, azygous, mesenteric, brachial, and crural veins but whether they had a function. If so, it was asked will it hamper the ebb and flow theory of Galen?

History

Credit for discovering the function of venous valves as one-way doors allowing the blood to flow in only one direction and preventing its regression goes to Fabricius ab Acquapendente (1533–1619).[9] He was selected to Chair the Department of Anatomy at the University of Padua on April 10, 1565, at a very early age of thirty-two years. Prior to his appointment this position had been vacant for two years.

It is contentious whether it is solely his discovery or there were other scientists who also noticed it during the same time. His student, William Harvey, was to become the most astute and most famous scientist in the history of medicine to follow. Harvey based his work on the discovery of his teacher, Fabricius, and unquestionably admitted its lineage. Later in the history Acquapendente solely inherited this credit. Even Fabricius did not refute Galen's theory for fear of losing recognition for his invention. He made compromises and accommodated Galen's concepts within the realm of his discovery. Harvey was exposed to and studied the function of the valves from his teacher even before he published his findings. Harvey's experiments rotated around the function of the valves as described in the previous chapter. Thus by the naked eye observation he was able to establish a new and true understanding of circulation. No wonder he was obsessed with the venous valves and in his entire monologue on the heart there is only one diagram depicting the venous valves of the forearm, which explains the various tourniquet tests he conducted on this basis. Retrospectively, these may appear to be simple experiments. However, it is the genius of Harvey that gave him an insight into circulation and ultimately concluded in his courageous declaration.

Reviewing the history of the venous valves as well as a review of my own experience, I am very much convinced and can make the statement, "The role that the venous valves played in the discovery of the mechanical function of the ventricular systole by Harvey and again 400 years later, inspired and directed me to discover the mechanical function of the atrial diastole." In the evolution of understanding of the mechanical function of the human heart and the laws governing the motion of blood in the circulatory system, the revelation of the role played by the ventricular chambers in Harvey's estimation and of the atrial chambers in the author's studies were inspiring and were revealed if at all by the venous valves and the interconnection of these events and will forever remain a mystery in history *chapter five*

Motion of blood in the venous system—novel findings

Velocity—a new parameter

The movement of blood is the dynamic inner manifestation and reflection of the presence of life in the human body. The physical character of the blood is a continuous flow in the arteries, capillaries, and veins. It is also the most important sign of life. Like any fluid, the laws that govern the flow are the same and apply to blood as well, even if it is flowing in a closed vacuum circuit. It moves from a higher pressure to a lower pressure. The only difference is in the arteries as they flow within a positive pressure and in the veins within a negative pressure system. Pressure is the force that blood exerts against the walls of the vessels as it moves. As a result of positive pressure in the arteries it is easily measured by a sphygmomanometer. It moves from the corresponding ventricle toward the peripheral systemic or pulmonary arteries. However, in the veins it is moving in collapsible tubes from a lower to a higher negative pressure and from the peripheral systemic or pulmonary veins into the corresponding atria. Ventricular systole is responsible for the motion of blood in the arteries. It slows down as it reaches the capillaries and it is slowest in the capillaries probably because it is located where all the exchange of gas and nutritional contents of the blood into the tissues occurs. Pressure is almost insignificant by the time blood leaves the capillaries and enters the venules. Blood flow in the veins is not the direct result of ventricular contraction as Sir William Harvey thought. According to present concepts as uncovered by this author, blood flows in the veins and back to the atrium primarily by atrial suction force during diastole. There are other adjunctive forces contributing to blood flow and they are skeletal muscle action, respiratory movements, and constriction of smooth muscles in the venous wall itself.

Blood pressure is the only parameter that we use to understand the hemodynamics of blood in the arteries at the present time. Technically, venous pressure cannot be measured by a sphygmomanometer. We have created a method to measure the weight of the column of the blood in the venous system and we consider it to be venous pressure in order to understand the venous hemodynamics. This is because pressure was the only age-old parameter by which we understood the hemodynamics. We have applied the same parameter when it comes to evaluating and treating diseases of the venous system.

During the 1970s and 1980s there was a renewed interest in the diagnosis and treatment of venous diseases. Limitations of the significance of measurement of venous pressure became very obvious in order to reflect the outcome of the new modalities of surgical procedures and treatment of chronic venous insufficiency disease (CVID). Conventional venous pressure measurement that was used to compare the preoperative and postoperative results or to understand the severity of venous insufficiency revealed its shortcomings as noted by researchers in the field of venous pressure. Raju[30] and Taheri[31] and colleagues added their own modifications of venous pressure testing to reflect the results of their methods of treatment. New tests were invented related to venous reflux and refilling time and many other variations of them.[31] During the early 1980s this author devised a below the knee vein valve transplantation as his method of treatment for CVID and in doing so he experienced the same dilemma. As a result, we decided to find a new parameter or new modality with which to study the venous hemodynamics. This was the first time an attempt was made to study the velocity of blood in the venous system directly.

The following method is described to measure that velocity, although it is not sophisticated it is not as crude as the first method used to measure blood pressure. This subject was definitely enlightened, heralding that it could be an important parameter of the future to understand the venous and arterial run in: hemodynamics. One might better appreciate it if it is described through the history of measuring blood pressure.

Reverend Stephen Hales in the year 1733 inserted a brass and glass tube into the carotid artery of his mare and noticed to his astonishment that the blood level rose in the tube to a height of 8 feet 3 inches. It was so high that it is said that to insert the last extension to the tube he worked out by climbing on the branch of a tree. When Hales coined the words blood pressure to identify this phenomenon, he was not aware that he had opened a new door to the understanding of hemodynamics. It took more than 150 years for the genius of Riva Rocci, Korotkoff, and Mohammed to design a sphygmomanometer to measure blood pressure by a non-invasive method based on the experiment of the Reverend Stephen Hales.

During the early part of the 20th century, Harvey Cushing introduced the sphygmomanometer for the clinical use in this country despite enormous resistance and criticism from the rest of the medical fraternity. Ever since then physicians have been dependent upon the measurement of pressure not only of the arteries but also of the veins in order to understand the hemodynamics during both the states of health and disease. The law that governs the motion of blood is the same in the venous and arterial systems. However, the conditions under which it moves in the venous system are totally different. Most of the time it has to move against the gravitational force, and it has to move in negative pressure tubes that are potentially collapsible. Hence the flow of blood from a higher to a lower positive pressure is not a quality of venous hemodynamics. However, physicians are still dependent upon the measurement of venous pressure to understand that of the venous hemodynamics. Despite its limitations there are no other better parameters available. Many modifications of venous pressure have been reported, each claiming to be better than the other, which is a natural outcome.

It is my hope that the unsophisticated method described by us to measure the velocity of venous blood will improve and not only that this test can measure the average velocity of blood in three areas of the vascular tree: they are the arteries, capillaries, and the venous system put together. I hope one day that velocity can be measured in each of the above systems separately just as we noted previously in the history of blood pressure and the crude method that was first discovered by literally bleeding an artery. This too later fell into the hands of three geniuses who were able to convert it into a simple tool that today has become the worldwide standard to measure blood pressure.

Objective

Since 1986, we have attempted an alternative method to understand venous hemodynamics in certain conditions by directly measuring the transit time of blood from a given point in the arterial tree to the desired point in the venous tree. This reflects the venous velocity of blood. This study was conducted in healthy individuals by recording the normal velocity and in those patients who were suffering from certain venous diseases.

Materials

This report includes fifteen studies conducted in ten individuals. Among them two normal individuals were studied as controls. In the remaining eight patients two studies were done on the same patient with CVID secondary to vein valve incompetence. This patient underwent vein valve transplantation and had both pre- and postoperative studies. These studies were done on patients with chronic obstructive venous disease. Two studies were done on patients with therapeutic arteriovenous (AV) fistulas, with the fistula between the superficial femoral artery and the great saphenous vein in the femoral triangle. Both were done to maintain a postoperative high venous outflow in the treatment of obstructive venous disease. One study was done on a patient with acute deep vein thrombosis (Table 5.1, #10). Another study was done on a patient with mixed etiology who had both occlusive arterial disease and incompetent valvular disease in the deep venous system. Among the above patients four studies were repeated for the following reasons. In one study there was extravasation of technetium following multiple attempts to inject it into the femoral artery. In another study an injection was made into the femoral vein instead. In two studies there were technical errors in the process of the gamma camera recording and the collection of data. All of the studies were repeated following an interval and an adequate time interval for the radioactivity of the initial injection to completely clear from the patient's body.

Table 5.1 Chronic Venous Insufficiency Disease

Studies	Etiology	t_1—Seconds
# 1	Control	22
# 2	Control	28
# 3	A.V. Fistula (therapeutic)	< 5
# 4	A.V. Fistula (therapeutic)	< 5
# 5	Mixed etiology	220
# 6	Venous Obstructive Disease	150
# 7	Venous Obstructive Disease	200
# 8	Venous Obstructive Disease	180
# 9	Acute Deep Vein Thrombosis	158
# 10	Vein Valve Incompetence Preoperative	256
# 11	Vein Valve Incompetence Postoperative	62

All of the patients including the normal individuals had the following noninvasive tests. They were segmental arterial Doppler pressure with ankle brachial index, maximum venous outflow, and venous capacitance tests, venous reflux test, and venous pressure measurement in the supine position and standing and exercising. All of the patients underwent ascending phlebography. All patients with the exception of one who had acute deep venous thrombosis (DVT) underwent descending phlebography. A diagnosis of venous disease was made in these patients based on ascending and descending phlebography. In addition, the patient with mixed etiology had a femoral angiogram.

Method

The patient was kept on a 45° semi-recumbent position by raising the head end of the table (Figure 5.1). All the tests were conducted with the patients in the same position. When the individual stands erect the gravitational force is at its peak and should create maximum resistance to the venous flow of blood toward the heart from the lower extremities. Hence the velocity of venous blood is theoretically at its lowest level. Under the present available technology this test cannot be performed with the patient standing up; therefore we opted for the semi-recumbent position. A number 25-gauge needle is attached to a

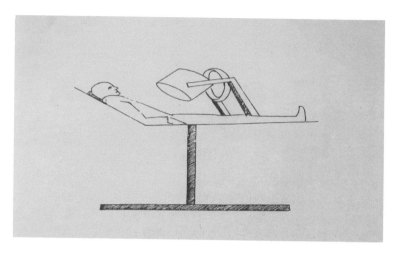

Figure 5.1 Semi-recumbent position of the patient at a 45° by raising the head end of the table.

short connecting tube (small bore extension tube) with a length of 8 inches priming volume: 0.4 mL (Byron Medical Inc.). The tube and needle are flushed with a normal heparin sodium chloride solution. The needle is inserted into the femoral artery of the leg to be tested. A sample of blood is withdrawn for arterial blood gas analysis to ensure that the needle is in the artery. Venous velocity is measured by the following method: 20 mCi of technetium 99 m in human serum albumin is with a 3 cc syringe and attached to the connecting tube. A gamma camera is adjusted to record the activity in the ipsilateral iliac vein (excluding the injection site). Technetium is injected as a single bolus. The gamma camera is started to coincide with the injection of technetium.

Data are acquired at 5-second intervals for a span of 5 minutes totaling 60 frames of recording (Figure 5.2). The data acquired are stored and processed by a computer. In each study gamma variant graphs were obtained. The time-activity curve (Figure 5.3) is generated by drawing the region of interest on the iliac vein of the same side. The t_1 is the time duration from the time of the injection into the femoral artery to the time of peak activity in the iliac vein on the same side.[32] Once the technetium reaches the general circulation that time activity curve continues as a plateau. The t_1 reflects the transit time of injected technetium directly related

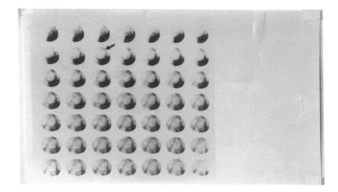

Figure 5.2 Gamma camera recording at 5-second interval. The arrow indicates the appearance of the left iliac vein. Notice as the time progresses that the radio-nuclear activity increases in the left vein and then reaches a plateau. Once radio-nuclear activity reaches systemic circulation both iliac veins are visible.

to the velocity of the flow of blood from the site of injection in the femoral artery through the entire arterial tree of that lower extremity and AV capillary shunt into the venous tree up to the ipsilateral iliac vein.

The test is conducted on all individuals under normal body temperature, cardiac rate, and blood pressure. It is done under

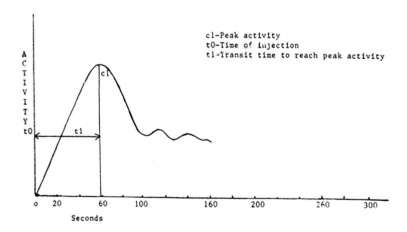

Figure 5.3 Diagrammatic explanation of time activity curve.

similar conditions and room temperature to minimize the above factors that influence body circulation during the study.

Findings

This study is done on normal individuals (Table 5.1, #1 and #2). They are young adults without any history of medical illness and with a normal ankle-brachial index. Maximum venous outflow, venous capacitance, and venous reflux studies were normal. For normal individuals the average circulation time recorded t_1 is 25 seconds (Figure 5.4). This reflects the velocity of venous blood in a healthy normal state. In patients #3 and #4 (Table 5.1) who underwent AV fistula for the treatment of venous occlusive disease both showed a t_1 of less than 5 seconds (Figure 5.5).

In these patients the peak activity of the iliac vein was instantaneously reached following injection to the common femoral artery. In #5 (Table 5.1) the t_1 is 220 seconds observed in the patient with mixed etiology. This patient had multilevel arterial disease with segmental occlusion of the superficial femoral and tibial arteries documented on femoral angiography. He also had venous valvular incompetency of the superficial and deep venous system that was documented on descending phlebography.

Three patients who had CVID secondary to chronic segmental venous obstructive disease had the following t_1: Patient #6 who is an athlete (a cyclist at the international level) had a deep

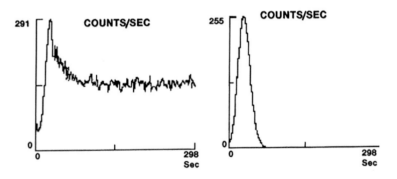

Figure 5.4 Gamma curve showing circulation time as t_1-28 seconds in a healthy individual (control study).

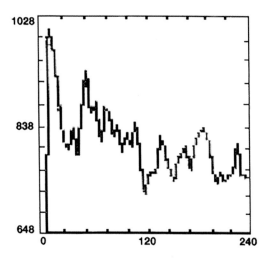

Figure 5.5 Circulation time recorded in a patient with therapeutic arteriovenous fistula between the femoral artery and the great saphenous vein. Note the per second activity reached in the ipsilateral iliac vein instantaneously (t_1 = <5 seconds).

venous obstruction involving the external iliac and femoral vein areas. The t_1 recorded in this patient is 150 seconds. Patient #7, an active football player at the college level, has a past history of drug injections to superficial veins and to the deep veins of the groin. This patient was found to have venous obstructive disease in the superficial venous system and right iliac venous segment and his t_1 was 200 seconds. Patient #8 had a past history of abdominal surgery (complicated appendicular abscess) and was found to have an isolated right iliac vein occlusion. The t_1 in this patient was 180 seconds. All patients had nonhealing ulcers on the ankle for more than 5 years with pain on the weight-bearing area and skin changes to the leg usually found in CVID. Patient #9 was admitted for acute deep vein thrombosis of the femoral segment and was found to have a t_1 of 158 seconds (Figure 5.6).

Figures 5.7 and 5.8 are two studies done on the same patient (#10 and #11). This patient was found to have deep venous valvular incompetency documented on descending phlebography. He had a nonhealing ankle ulcer for 15 years with a past history of ligation and stripping of the superficial venous system. He underwent

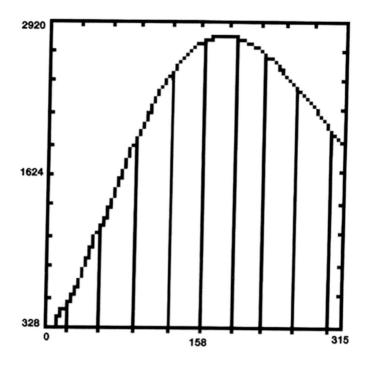

Figure 5.6 Circulation time t_1 is 158 seconds in a patient with acute deep venous thrombosis of the right leg involving the superficial femoral and popliteal vein segments.

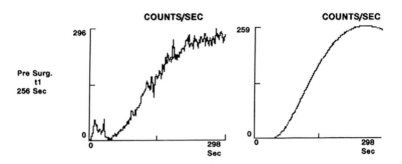

Figure 5.7 Preoperative study on a patient with deep venous valvular incompetency. Preoperative t_1 is 256 seconds.

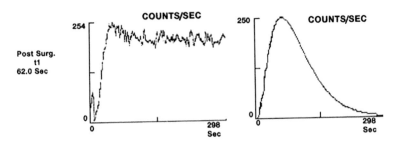

Figure 5.8 Postoperative study on the same patient after below the knee vein valve transplantation. Postoperative t_1 is 62 seconds.

vein valve transplantation below the knee popliteal segment by this author's technique.[17] In this patient (Figure 5.7) pre- and postoperative (Figure 5.8) studies were done. Preoperative t_1 was 256 seconds and postoperative t_1 was 62 seconds. The tests were uneventful in all patients.

Discussion

t_1 records the transit time of technetium or the circulation time of blood beginning at the injection site of the femoral artery and ending at the selected site of the ipsilateral iliac vein. Although blood has a different velocity as it traverses to the arterial capillary and venous segment of its passage, t_1 represents the average velocity. Among the patients studied there was only one patient with mixed etiology in whom the velocity was decreased by both arterial and venous disease. The remaining patients had normal arterial circulation as documented by the ankle-brachial index. The prolonged t_1 was caused by decreased velocity of the blood in the venous segment of its passage.

The patient with venous valvular incompetency (VVI) recorded a slight fall in the ankle brachial index (ABI). Postoperative t_1 was recorded and compared under the same ABI. In patients with VVI, the incompetent venous valves to the affected areas of the venous tree allowed a retrograde flow of blood resulting in a private venous circulation and thereby causing an overall decrease in the velocity of the venous circulation and as a result in a prolonged circulation time t_1. This same patient had a single vein valve transplantation to the popliteal vein segment below the knee by the method described by this author. Postoperatively this patient showed a significant decrease in t_1 reflecting an increase in venous blood velocity. Following surgery, the transplanted competent venous valve prevented retrograde flow of the venous blood and thereby stopped private venous circulation in the diseased leg. This increased venous velocity following vein valve transplantation. This patient had a 15-year history of a nonhealing ankle ulcer and pain with all the skin changes associated with CVID. In this patient the ulcer completely healed in five weeks with primary epithelialization of the skin and symptomatic relief of pain. The remaining skin changes stayed the same. This patient's t_1 did not decrease to the normal level but there was considerable decrease of t_1 toward the normal level suggesting an increase in venous blood velocity. As a result, this led to a new question. Is normalization of velocity of the blood in the circulatory system a key factor in the supply of nutrients and oxygen to tissue that results in wound healing and spontaneous epithelialization? Venous pressure studies of this patient are reported in Table 5.1 and studies #10 and #11. In chronic obstructive venous disease and acute DVT venous blood has to take a circulatory route through collaterals to reach the iliac vein. This causes an overall decrease in venous blood velocity resulting in prolonged circulation time t_1. Venous blood velocity is at its peak in patients with a therapeutic AV fistula which is created between the superficial femoral artery and the common femoral vein. An injection is carried out proximal to the AV fistula and peak radioactivity is reached in the cephalad iliac vein instantaneously. This does not reflect the velocity of blood in the lower extremity venous tree distal to the fistula.

Conclusion

Most of the parameters used today to understand the venous hemodynamics are directly or indirectly related to pressure. In certain disease conditions there are subtle changes that take place in hemodynamics continuously in the human body and that may not reflect any change in the venous or arterial pressures. In such situations physicians are completely at a loss to understand the ongoing events of patients. CVID is one such situation in the venous system. A patient in a state of shock or in cardiac arrest in which no arterial pressures can be recorded are classic examples of inadequacies of dependency on pressure monitoring of the arterial system.

Arterial pressure is dependent upon positive pressure measurement and applicable only to the arterial limb of the circulatory system. In the venous limb circulation is in collapsible tubes and operated by negative pressure. The circulatory system consists of the heart and arterial, capillary, and venous limbs and they operate as one system. A common parameter has to be found and used to understand the hemodynamics of the whole system. This study is an attempt to find an alternative parameter applicable to the whole system as circulation of blood is the sign of life and its main functional feature. Maintaining a particular average velocity in the whole system is a necessity for the "milieu interior" of the body and is dependent upon a coordinated function of all four limbs. Understanding this aspect and getting a grip on the measurement of velocity as a parameter to know the changes in hemodynamics can help in the diagnosis, treatment, and prognosis of the various diseases of cardiac, arterial, capillary, and venous origin. It also may be an important parameter of the future. This study is based on the direct measurement of velocity of the blood, which may prove to be a better parameter in the future and open new doors in this direction.

chapter six

Venous flow is pulsatile

When the ventricle contracts it surges a volume of blood into the great arteries. The arteries expand as a result of this volume of blood which can be manually felt and visually observed. We have termed this phenomenon the arterial pulse. Historically, in the circulatory system the contraction of the heart or of the vessels was named "systole" and the dilatation or filling phase was called "diastole." The term diastole was also applied to the pulsation of the arteries during that phase. Currently the terms systole and diastole are restricted to the description of the atria and ventricles of the heart. Dilatation or diastole of the artery is now termed "pulsation." However, the age-old theory that the systole is the only active phase of the heart remains unchanged. The diastole is always considered to be the resting phase, wherein the supplying of the cardiac chambers with blood occurs during this phase.

During ventricular systole there is a surge of blood into the arterial system which increases the flow and volume of the blood in the arteries. During the diastole of the ventricle the arteries do not completely collapse owing to the compliance in the wall of the artery. This helps the circulation in two ways. First if the arteries were to completely collapse during diastole then there would have been cessation of the flow of blood to the arteries. This would have resulted in the doubling of the workload on the consecutive ventricular systole. Second, compliance of the artery keeps the blood in motion during diastole, permitting the consecutive ventricular systole to take over the flow of blood in the already dilated arteries and resulting in a decrease of the workload of the ventricle by half. This observation of ventricular systole with active contraction of the muscles pushing the blood into the arteries and refilling itself during diastole without any interference in the flow of blood in the arteries has resulted in the popular inferences that systole is the only active function in the cardiac cycle of the heart and diastole, which is the filling phase, is the resting phase of the heart.

DOI: 10.1201/b22792-6

This author has convincingly proved that both systole and diastole are equally active phases of the cardiac cycle and contribute equally to the function of the heart. This is because during both phases there are chemical, physical, and electrical changes taking place at the cellular level. This author has experimentally proved both contraction and dilatation of cardiac muscle as active phenomena and both are not the resting phase of the cardiac cycle. At the present time we can say if at all the heart rests, then it is for a moment during the intervals between the systole and diastole. This resting is in the sense that consumption of energy is lowest by the heart in that intermediate phase.

The systolic phase of the ventricle is instrumental in increasing the flow rhythmically in the arterial system resulting in rhythmic pulsation of the arteries. However in the venous system there are no visible or palpable pulsations observed, as the ventricular systole has no effect on the flow of blood in the veins. In addition, the veins are collapsible tubes and there is no effect of the ventricular systole on the venous circulation. When Sir William Harvey established that the arteries and veins are in continuity and form a closed system, he was of the opinion that the ventricular force continuously pushes the blood in this closed circuit and is responsible for the motion of blood both in the arteries and the venous system. Harvey gave credit to the presence of the venous valves as one-way doors in the venous system, thus permitting blood to flow toward the heart and prevent back flow. The function of the valves was taught to him by his mentor and professor Fabricius Hieronymous Acquapendente. As a result of this fact, Harvey concluded that both in the arterial and venous system blood flows as a result of ventricular systolic force.

Subsequent researchers after Harvey realized that ventricular systolic contraction only produces enough force to push the blood in the arteries until it reaches the capillaries, beyond which it has no effect. Yet they were at a loss to explain the main force that keeps the blood in motion in the venous system. Various other adjunctive forces were described as discussed in previous chapters. If left alone for ventricular systolic force, blood would cease to flow beyond the capillary level and would result in stagnation in the venous system. At present it is thought that the motion of blood in the veins is linear. Following the experimental evidence that the atrial diastole creates a negative pressure and thereby activates the flow of blood in the great veins, just like the ventricular systolic force activates the flow of blood in the arterial system resulting in arterial pulsatile motion of blood. We decided to make a series of experimental observations and collect the data on the effects of atrial diastole on the motion of blood in the great veins.

Method

We gathered data from the experiments done on mongrel canines. We developed an experimental model similar to the model that we did for the recording of the function of the atrial diastole. During the entire experiment the canine was kept in the erect position so as to have the gravitational force affect the venous flow. Separate catheters were inserted into the right atrium, inferior vena cava, and femoral artery. Each one was connected to a pressure monitor through the transducer. Whatever changes that occurred in the right atrium, inferior vena cava, and femoral artery were recorded by each monitor with simultaneous graphic tracing and hard copy recording.

Electrocardiographic (EKG) leads were applied, and simultaneous EKG tracings were taken during the entire experiment (Figure 6.1). A cross-clamp was used to occlude the superior vena cava. Pressure changes reflected in graphic tracing were very obvious in the femoral artery and right atrium. The graphic changes that occurred in the flow of blood in the inferior vena cava were very subtle and required careful observation. Nevertheless, there were rhythmic changes occurring in relation to each cardiac cycle. In the inferior vena cava recording one can notice a rhythmic curve. The tip of the curve of the graph is flat and wide; it has an anachronic notch and a dicrotic notch with a flat top. It is comparatively more prominent and is particularly enhanced when the superior vena cava is cross-clamped.

Now let us study and compare each graphic tracing and try to determine what phase of the atrial cycle in which it occurs in the inferior vena cava. We can infer the cardiac activity from the EKG of the canine. The changes occurring in the femoral flow depicted by the anachronic part of the graphic wave concur with the QRST-wave in the EKG suggesting there is an increased flow of blood in the artery during ventricular systole. The graphic tracing that

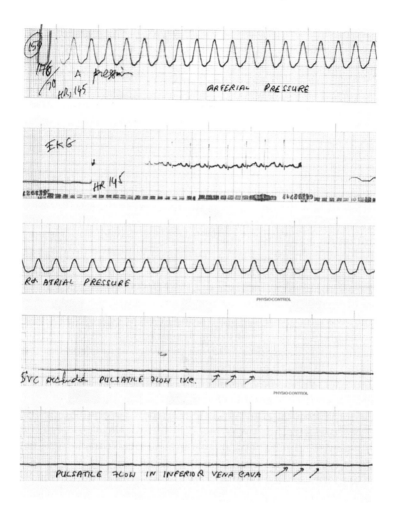

Figure 6.1 Electrocardiographic leads applied with simultaneous EKG tracings during the entire experiment. The above diagram indicates the various graphic tracings from above and downward. The first graphic tracing records changes in the femoral arterial pressure. That is picked by the catheter and inserted into the femoral artery of the canine followed by the EKG tracing. The third graphic tracing immediately below the EKG records the pressure changes occurring in the right atrial chamber. The fourth graphic tracing records the flow changes in the inferior vena cava when the superior vena cava is totally occluded. The fifth and bottom graphic tracing is the flow changes that are occurring in the inferior vena cava without the occlusion of the superior vena cava.

occurs in the atrial chamber concurs with the ascending curve of the P-waves in the EKG, suggesting the diastolic phase of the right atrium.[29] The graphic curve noticed in the inferior vena cava occurring rhythmically concurs with the P-waves of the EKG during the atrial diastole of the right atrium. This suggests that there is an increased motion of the column of blood in the inferior vena cava during each diastole of the right atrium and that is why it is rhythmic with the atrial diastole. We have already experimentally proved that the atrial diastole creates negative pressure and applies suction force to the venous blood that is present in the great veins (superior and inferior vena cava) and that directly drain into the atrial chamber. The column of blood in the superior and inferior vena cavas in the immediate vicinity of the right atrium moves into the atrial chamber causing the filling of the atrium during diastole. In the inferior vena cava` it has to move against the gravitational force especially when the body is in the erect position. During each diastole a certain volume of blood from the vena cava empties into the atria, thereby creating an empty space in the upper-most column of the great veins. This is immediately filled by the subsequent column of blood below and adjacent to it, setting up the motion of blood in the venous tree and creating a rippling phenomenon along the entire column of blood in the venous tree. So there occurs a motion of blood during atrial diastole in the entire venous tree. During atrial systole there is a weakening of the force and the motion temporarily slows until the next cycle of the atrial diastole takes over. This creates a rhythmic motion of blood in the venous tree. The motion of the blood in the venous system is rhythmic and increases and decreases in a pulsatile manner and is not linear as presently has been thought.

This experimental recording of the data confirms that the motion of blood in the veins is rhythmical and waxes and wanes, as it is pulsatile.

## chapter seven

Motion of venous valves in humans—a new discovery

History of modern medicine

In modern medicine history when one peruses the subject of venous disease, it is found that Frederick Adolph Trendelenburg (1840–1924) makes an unforgettable contribution. Upon ocular observation and manual tests, Trendelenburg was able to describe in detail the etiology of varicose veins and discover a surgical procedure to treat them. During the ensuing next one hundred years not much progress was made in the field of venous disease.

On the basis of Trendelenburg's theory, stripping and ligation of the great or short saphenous veins of the lower extremities became part of the surgical treatment for venous insufficiency.[1,2] Stripping and ligation were once the most common surgical procedures practiced in hospitals.

As surgeons became more involved in diseases and the treatment of arterial system, the diseases of the venous system were dumped on the back shelf. Many maladies pertaining to the venous system such as chronic venous ulcers, venous insufficiency, and post-thrombotic syndromes were not adequately treated. The management of venous ulcers was insufficiently addressed by the scholars of the upper medical hierarchical system. This resulted in patients who were suffering from terminal end-stage venous insufficiency from intractable ulcers. The only treatment performed on those patients was that of wound cleaning and dressing each time the patient visited the clinic, and it was generally carried out by interns at the beginning of their surgical training.

DOI: 10.1201/b22792-7

Management of venous disorders

In the 1970s the surgical fraternity showed a noteworthy redevelopment in the management of venous disorders and addressed problems of the venous system.

It was around the same time that Kistner in 1971 performed a valvuloplasty to correct the retrograde leaking of the femoral venous valves in the treatment for venous insufficiency caused by valvular incompetency.[14] This procedure generated much interest and Dr. Sheshadri Raju popularized it. Dr. Syed Taheri performed the first vein valve transplant in the femoral vein and in 1984 this author performed the first vein valve transplant in the popliteal vein below the knee.[15]

Author's personal experience

At the beginning of my vascular surgery practice in 1980 at the Brooklyn Jewish Medical Center, which was a 940-bed hospital, there were many senior well-known cardiothoracic surgeons. As the most junior vascular surgeon it was difficult for me to obtain vascular referrals. Therefore out of necessity my interest turned toward those patients with venous ulcers.

During those days venous duplex machines were still primordial, so I personally began performing descending venous phlebography to evaluate venous valvular incompetency in patients with chronic venous disease and those who were suffering from leg ulcers around the ankle. Originally the technique of descending phlebography was described by Tore Sylvan in 1950. He performed this procedure by cannulating the femoral vein with an open cut down.[10] This procedure was further simplified by Dr. Taheri. He performed a blind percutaneous puncture of the brachial vein under local anesthesia and advanced the catheter under fluoroscopy to the desired femoral vein to perform descending phlebography. He was a brilliant surgeon and inventor and I had an opportunity to interact with him personally during those early days. I preferred to do all my descending phlebography by blind percutaneous puncture of the right internal jugular vein and to advance the catheter under fluoroscopy into the desired femoral vein. I also innovated a new method of using a balloon catheter with a double lumen to advance it beyond the venous valves in a retrograde fashion without causing damage to the valves using a guidewire.[13] This was the first retrograde catheterization devised in the venous tree. Later it was given a US patent (February 26, 1991 patent #4,995,878), and new catheters were made by the company, Ideas for Medicine, at that time. This was useful before sophisticated duplex scanners were introduced. These catheters and the technique were also used for retrograde venous embolectomies. These procedures were done by the author in the radiology suite with the help of an assistant resident and a radiology technician. The procedure was performed under fluoroscopy using a tilt table. The tip of the catheter was placed in line with the pubic tubercle, which is a surface marking for femoral vein valves. Then the table was tilted to the semi-erect position and contrast medium was injected. Fluoroscopic recordings were taken to evaluate the competency of the valves. Incompetent valves allowed retrograde flow of the contrast material downward in the venous tree. During one such early procedure around 1984 I experienced an accidental event when for the first time I noticed the motion of the venous valves. This is already narrated in the previous chapter.

I also read an immense amount of literature on this subject from the time of Hippocrates to the present day. But previously there was no mention anywhere in the past or present literature about the motion of the venous valves. Therefore I decided to investigate in detail the motion of venous valves in humans. I began by observing the motion of the venous valves in each patient as I was performing a descending phlebography and I recorded the events with cine recording.

Methods

The data were collected by performing the following procedure.[16] The procedure was performed in the X-ray suite under fluoroscopy on a tilt table under local anesthesia. An 18-gauge angio-catheter was introduced into the right internal jugular vein and through that a guidewire 0.032 inches in diameter and then advanced to the area of the right femoral vein. Along the guidewire, using the Seldinger technique a number 6-F size 100-cm-long catheter was introduced into the femoral vein. The guidewire was removed and the contrast medium was injected with a 60 mL syringe in small doses of 10 mL each. The motion in the form of opening and closing of these valves and their relationship to the cardiac cycle and postures were recorded in more than 150 patients.

A study made on a 67-year-old black male is presented in this chapter. The motion was recorded while the patient was in a recumbent position (flat on his back) and then in an 80 degrees semi-erect position. The continuous cine recording consists of 12 frames. Recording time of each frame and its number is automatically included in each exposure. The photos presented are the reduced copies from 8 × 12 inches of original X-rays. As the time of exposure and frame number are not easily visible in the reduced photograph of the original X-ray films it is separately written on each photo. In Figure 7.1 frame 119 begins at 15 hours 52 minutes and the last phase of the 31st second. In Figure 7.2 frame 130 ends at the middle phase of the 34th second and runs for approximately 2.75 seconds. During the time femoral venous valves open exactly four times (check frame numbers 119, 122, 126, 129) and close three times (check frame numbers 121, 124, 127) (Figures 7.1 and 7.3).

Results

The X-ray shows the valves in the common femoral, superficial femoral, profunda femoris, and great saphenous venous segments. These valves open and close in synchrony with each cardiac cycle during atrial diastole. They are timed with the electrocardiogram recording of the individual. He has 69 heart beats and the valves open and close 69 times per minute. The patient is kept in the erect posture. The tip of the catheter seen in the right femoral vein is introduced through the right internal jugular vein.

These venous valves open and close in synchronized rhythm to each cardiac cycle. The motion of the valves is least obvious while the subject is lying down and becomes very prominent when he is in the erect posture. X-rays above show a continuous cine recording of this motion. The first frame in the figure is numbered 119 and the last one is 130 for a total of 12 frames. Recording of each frame is timed. Frame 119 begins at 15:52:31 (hours:min:seconds) and frame 130 ends at 15:52:34. Whole recording run time is close to 2.75 seconds. In a little less than 3 seconds the femoral valves open four times and close three times. All these valves open and close simultaneously. A constant and rhythmic motion occurred during each cardiac cycle. This is better seen

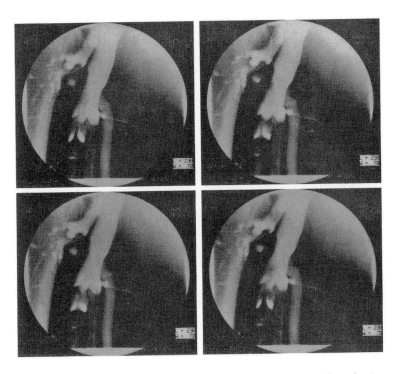

Figure 7.1 Continuous cine recording of the femoral vein valves during the injection of the contrast material. This has four frames recorded in sequence. Each X-ray records the frame number at the right upper corner and the time of record at the lower left corner. Frame 119 upper left at the 15th hour and 52nd minute and the last phase of the 31st second shows complete opening of the valves. Closure of the valves begins at frame number 120 upper right and completes in 121 lower left. Frame number 122 lower right shows opening of the valves.

and appreciated in the videotape recording done simultaneously (now available on You Tube under *"New Discovery: Motion of the Venous Valves in Human Beings"* (https://youtube.be/7XjddZYLp).

Discussion

A review of the past literature that contains reference to the valves in the veins of human beings goes back to the days of venesection practiced by Hippocrates in the treatment of various illnesses[28]

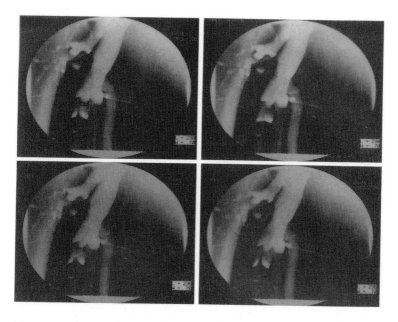

Figure 7.2 Frame 127 shows complete closure of the valves and frame 129 shows complete opening of the valves. Frame number 130 ends at the 15th hour 52nd minute, and middle of the 34th second.

and is traced to the present time.[28] However, there is no mention of the motion of venous valves in any form by any author at any time.[18,19] That is why the present finding is new. The motion of the venous valves was noticed in these individuals. In some individuals it is very obvious and in some it is subtle, but it is always present when carefully looked for. It becomes more prominent when the test is done in the erect posture. This is also noticeable in duplex scanning of the femoral and popliteal veins. This chapter describes the recording of motion of venous valves occurring during each cardiac cycle. The above findings on the motion of valves was made approximately 400 years after Fabricius made the discovery that these valves are one-way doors that allow the blood to flow in one direction toward the heart. This understanding during the time of William Harvey led him to unravel the mechanical function of the ventricles of the heart. Whether this motion is primarily inherent in the valves or is secondary to other forces

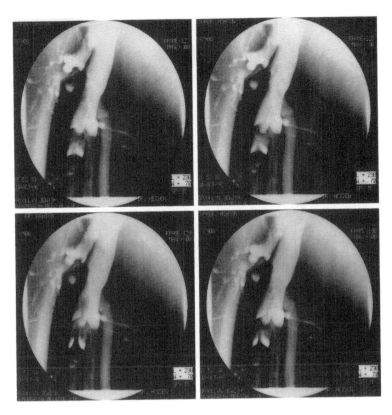

Figure 7.3 Frame 124 shows complete closure of the valve. Frame 126 shows complete opening of the valve.

and what is its relationship to the heart are questions that need to be addressed in the future.

In summary, this chapter records a discovery that venous valves in human beings open and close during each cardiac cycle in a rhythmical fashion. The motion is present in all postures but becomes more prominent when the person is in the erect posture. This chapter does not address whether this motion is passive or active or its relationship to heart function. This finding raises many questions related to venous circulation. It may provide a new understanding of the forces related to the motion of blood in the venous system.

Conclusion

We wanted to know if this motion was in relation to the heart. Therefore we began to simultaneously record the EKGs of patients during each procedure and tried to time it. Depolarization of the ventricle gives rise to the QRS complex and this main event demonstrated on the EKG machine by a blinking light and beeping sound occurring at the peak of T-waves and easy to time. Hence we were able to time the opening of the venous valve to the exact segment of the EKG recording and thereby associate the valvular motion with a particular part of the cardiac cycle. We observed that the opening of the venous valves coincides each time after the beeping or after the ventricular systole and before the beginning of the P-waves, clearly showing a relationship with the atrial diastole.

Author's reflection

Since this accidental discovery of the motion of venous valves I grew more and more restless as days passed. This entire phenomenon posed an enigma to me. I began to contemplate this subject, wondering if this was a new discovery or if it had been reported in past medical literature, and thus I began to research this subject. Up until that point in time it was my understanding that the venous valves gained importance only after recent significance reported by the etiology of the post-thrombotic syndrome and the varicose veins.

It took a movement of a group of surgeons to correct the incompetence of the valves by means of valvuloplasty or valve transplant as a newly evolved treatment method. My research gradually pulled me to the history of venous valves from the time of Hippocrates and Aristotle to the present day, which I have shared in the past chapters.

I note that the present observation of the motion of venous valves was never mentioned in the past literature and had become a new discovery on this subject. We have witnessed the mysterious role it played in the revelations of the secrets of the heart and the laws governing the motion of blood in the arterial system. When I began observing this in each patient undergoing descending phlebography the most beleaguering question in my mind was is this motion passive or active? It was so rhythmic and occurred during each cardiac cycle that it moved me to accept that it is connected to some phase of the cardiac cycle. I was able to record and time it with an EKG on the patient. The opening of the valves was occurring at the start of the P-waves, which coincided with atrial diastole. It was doubtless connected to the atrial diastole. However, it was very hard to explain the connection between the functionless atrial diastole and the opening of the valves.

Since the time of Aristotle the atrial chambers of the heart had no significance both anatomically and physiologically. As a matter of fact, during that era and up to the time of Galen the atrial chambers did not even exist as part of the heart but rather they were described as extensional pouches of the vena cava coming out of the liver. The same concept pertaining to the anatomy of the heart was also entertained by Harvey since he studied the *Anatomy of the Heart* written by these authors of the past. Even after the work of William Harvey they were considered functionless, particularly the diastolic phase of the heart which was considered to be the resting phase and functionless with the exception that they are a blood collecting tank of the heart. Coincidently, present-day thoughts and teaching have not changed.

Our understanding of the function of the muscle was based on the famous experiment and work of Ernest Henry Starling, a celebrity British physiologist of his generation.[20] His historical experiment on a frog's thigh became part of the curriculum of physiology for all medical students to conduct in the laboratory. We ran an electrical current into the thigh muscle and excited it in order to record the graphic tracing of the sudden contraction of the frog's thigh muscle. This experiment established that the muscle functions by contraction and is the active motion. Regaining its original status or length is by recoiling back to its original status, which is presumed to be a passive motion. This was inculcated in our minds and as students and this experiment resulted in such deep-rooted impressions (in our minds) and concluded that when muscles only contract and recoil back like a spring to a stretched state is passive and is the normal resting period. As of this result I have been unable to recognize the importance of the atrial diastole when the muscles were supposed to be regaining their resting phase of stretching immediately following the systolic phase of contraction.

This led me to develop an experimental model in the canine's heart and to study the atrial diastole in detail. Ultimately I was able to develop a model in which I could isolate the atrial chambers both functionally and physiologically and conduct a series of experiments. I shall share with you the outcome of these experimental studies. It took me a few years to interpret the data collected and a few more years to understand the interconnection between each event, interpret it, and offer an explanation. I had to make a shift in my basic thinking created by the popular teaching of the laws of motion of blood dependent upon the systolic phase of the ventricle as per Sir William Harvey and the laws of muscle contraction as established by Ernest Henry Starling, two of the most notable minds of the past. Ultimately I was able to realign my thinking, making a paradigm shift from the past and jumping out of the box under the dawning of the new light of understanding on the laws of muscle function of the heart, enabling me to interpret the collected data and the interconnected findings like a jigsaw puzzle. I presented these new findings in national and international forums. After many such presentations and many rejections of manuscripts for publication in peer review journals I enthusiastically continued my efforts despite the initial disappointments. Twenty-three years after my first presentation in 2013 I published my research in the *International Journal of Angiology,* and I shall present it as it is published in the journal.[21]

chapter eight

The dynamic function of the atrial diastole of the heart

This study demonstrates the dynamic function of the atrial diastole for the first time in the history of medicine following the revelation of ventricular function by Sir William Harvey. This study consists of two parts. The first part is the study of humans and the discovery of the rhythmic opening and closing of venous valves in the femoral vein segment during each cardiac cycle under fluoroscopy. Its relationship to the right atrial diastole is discussed in the previous chapter. The second part is an experimental model developed in a canine's heart. Experiments are conducted with the subjects in an erect posture in which the right atrium is partially and totally isolated physically and/or functionally. The right atrium was found to function as a suction pump and was readily demonstrated on graphic curves as a reaction and a reflex stretching of muscle fibers of the empty atrium. This creates considerable negative pressure during diastolic function and is responsible for venous return to the heart. Motive forces in the venous return are common knowledge in the present medical literature but are limited to respiration and skeletal muscle contraction of the extremities. The discovery of the right atrium as a suction force due to active and reflex stretching of muscle fibers during diastolic function thereby creating negative pressure represents a departure from the currently accepted paradigm established by Sir William Harvey (1576–1652) that the heart is an organ functioning solely by contraction of its ventricular chambers. This is the first time since then that a fundamental new discovery concerning cardiac mechanical function has been made utilizing experimental evidence.

For more than 1,300 years Galen's views (130–201 AD) dominated medical opinion and entire generations of physicians were unquestioning obedient students of his teaching. That is the

DOI: 10.1201/b22792-8

reason why the entry of Sir William Harvey (1574–1652 AD) into the medical world became such an important event in the history of modern medicine.

Galen observed that all ingested nutrition enters the gastrointestinal system and is transformed into blood draining from the intestines to the liver, from which it is distributed to various parts of the body. Hence he preached that the liver is the main organ of circulation. Harvey's life-long experiments on various animal hearts ultimately resulted in the following discoveries, which remain unchanged to this day.[22] They include:

1. The heart is the center of circulation.
2. Ventricles are the forward pushing pumps and provide the force to keep the blood in motion in the human body.
3. Circulation is a continuous phenomenon and not optional as thought until then. Blood leaves the ventricles and comes back to the atrium, moving in a circular fashion within the body.
4. Circulation is a closed-circuit system and the arteries and veins are interconnected.
5. It is the same volume of blood that circulates again and again.

However both Galen and Harvey did not understand one of the most important functions of blood, which was to carry oxygen from the lungs to various parts of the body and carbon dioxide from tissue back to the lungs.

Harvey had not discussed any functional role of the atria. It was not until later that anatomists identified that there are two additional chambers of the heart. These were considered passive and as the collecting chambers of the heart where venous blood returns and pools. Harvey thought the forward pushing force of the ventricles was adequate enough to keep blood in motion within the arteries and veins and return it to the atria.

Some of Harvey's opinions were later questioned. It has been voiced that the force imparted by the ventricles to the ejected blood is not sufficient to explain the venous return to the atria. The nature of other forces that may have contributed to the venous return has been a matter of heated discussion for centuries. At present two of the forces in the human body that play an important role in the motion of venous blood have been well established. The first is the skeletal muscle contraction, which is primarily the calf muscle pump and is known as the peripheral heart.[23] The second is from Bollinger who in 1971 clearly established the role of respiration in the circulation of blood.[24] The force responsible for venous return to the atria has not been explained. Scientists preceding Harvey as well as those following him theorized the forces contributing to the motion of blood under the broad headlines of *vis-a-tergo* (a force from the back by ventricular systole) and *vis-a-fronte* (a force from the front by ventricular diastole). None of these scientists, however, gave credit to diastolic dilatation of the atrial chambers of the heart.[25]

In reviewing past literature, only Wedemyer's[26] concept alluded to the idea of auricular dilatation that causes an aspirating effect on venous blood. With no experimental evidence backing this hypothesis, Donders[26] soon discarded it. In the book *Human Physiology* by Houssay[27] it is mentioned that during ventricular contraction intra-auricular pressure falls, having a slight aspirating effect on blood from the veins. Houssay states that it has little or no functional significance. It always had been thought that systole of the ventricles and atria is caused by contraction of muscle fibers and is considered to be active and dynamic and that the diastole was always thought to be the phase of relaxation. The present concept of motion of blood in the human body is illustrated in Chapter 3, Figure 3.2.

Description

Ventricular systolic force pushes the blood forward into the arteries. This force is exhausted by the time it reaches the capillaries. Blood is thought to move in the veins back into the atrium by respiration and peripheral muscular contraction. At present the atrium is considered only a passive receptacle and the heart is just a forward pushing pump.

Study on canines

Experiments were conducted on five mongrel canines with an average weight of 55 lb. Because gravitational force plays a role in the atrial function canines were kept in a semi-upright or upright position. Following intubation we administered general anesthesia to each canine and placed each one in a horizontal position on a wooden board that was rectangular in shape and with sideboards for the upper and lower extremities. Monitoring lines were placed, including a femoral arterial line for the continuous monitoring of arterial pressure with graphic tracing. A catheter was inserted through the jugular vein and into the right atrium and was connected to a pressure monitor through a transducer to record the atrial pressure changes during the experiment. An electrocardiographic machine was used for continuous EKG monitoring. Experiment I was conducted in all canines. Experiment II was conducted in the same canine several times and recorded the same finding.

Experiment III was conducted in two canines. Experiment IV was conducted in two canines.

Experiment I.

Forces were established contributing to the motion of venous blood and were neutralized utilizing the following method. We paralyzed the canine with muscle relaxants to prevent any contraction including even the twitching of skeletal muscles during this experiment. In doing so this excluded the muscular contraction aiding the venous flow in the body. A vertical midline incision was made from the xiphoid notch to the pubic tubercle keeping the thoracic and abdominal cavities open. We then transected the diaphragm with an anterior-posterior incision toward the vertebral column. In doing so this excluded the changes in the intrathoracic and intra-abdominal cavity pressure from contributing to venous blood flow by respiration. The wooden board with the canine was tilted upward and kept against the wall of the room. This kept the canine in an erect position during the rest of this experiment.

Experiment I was done in all five canines as a preliminary step. Figure 8.1 shows (a) the EKG indicating the sinus rhythm with a cardiac rate of 124/minute; (b) the beginning of the graphic curve recording the pressure in the right atrium as 7/-2 mmHg pressure. A catheter is then advance to the right ventricle. Of note is the increased height of the graphic curve and the rising pressure to 25/6 mmHg. The catheter was then withdrawn from the right atrium resulting in the restoration of the graphic curve and a pressure of 7/-2 mmHg. This experimental maneuver assured

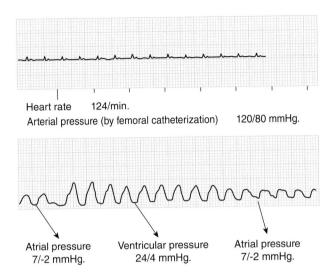

Heart rate   124/min.
Arterial pressure (by femoral catheterization)   120/80 mmHg.

Atrial pressure   Ventricular pressure   Atrial pressure
7/-2 mmHg.   24/4 mmHg.   7/-2 mmHg.

Figure 8.1 Experiment I. Continuous and simultaneous recording of three monitors. The upper graph is the EKG (the heart rate of the model is 124/min). Femoral arterial pressure is recorded as 120/80 mmHg. The lower graph is the model's right atrial pressure. The catheter is deliberately pushed from the right atrium to the right ventricle. It is brought back and affixed to the right atrium. The right atrial diastolic pressure is –2 mmHg.

the placement of the catheter in the right atrium during the remainder of the experiment. This maneuver was also utilized for each of the subsequent experiments with the catheter fixed in the right atrium.

Experiment II. Position of the Canine® Upright Experiment Clamping of the Superior Vena Cava

In Experiment II done in two canines (Figure 8.2) the canine is maintained at a 60° erect position. In this experiment changes of the right atrial pressure were studied by partial exclusion of the atria, ligating the superior vena cava using umbilical tapes over a Rommel clamp. We recorded the immediate changes. The arterial pressure progressively began to fall within a few seconds and threatened to reach a nonrecordable level if the experiment continued. Meanwhile

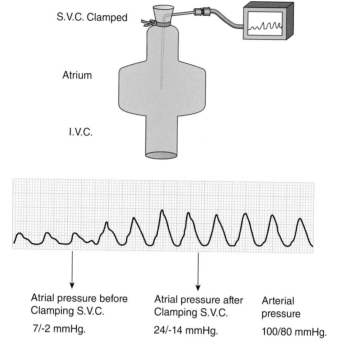

Figure 8.2 Experiment II. The superior vena cava is ligated and the atrial venous return is partially cut off. This results in an immediate fall of atrial diastolic negative pressure up to a –14 mmHg increase.

the graphic tracing in the right atria demonstrated a remarkable change by increasing three times in size, with a negative pressure reaching –14 mmHg. At this stage the experiment was discontinued by relaxing the ligature on the superior vena cava due to a rapid fall in arterial pressure.

Experiment III.

In Experiment III, done in two canines (Figure 8.3), the right atrium was totally excluded by simultaneously ligating both the superior and inferior vena cavas utilizing the same technique as described above. The immediate observation was indicated within a few seconds of ligation. The arterial pressure reached a nonrecordable level and the atrial chamber went into fibrillation. When we continued the experiment

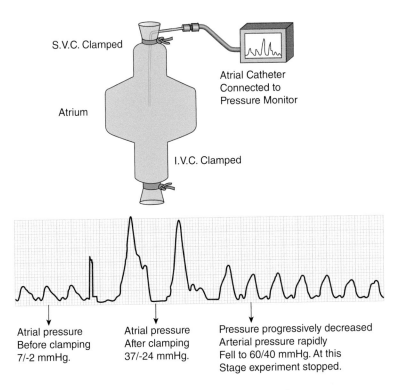

S.V.C. Clamped

Atrium

Atrial Catheter
Connected to
Pressure Monitor

I.V.C. Clamped

Atrial pressure
Before clamping
7/-2 mmHg.

Atrial pressure
After clamping
37/-24 mmHg.

Pressure progressively decreased
Arterial pressure rapidly
Fell to 60/40 mmHg. At this
Stage experiment stopped.

Figure 8.3 Experiment III. Both the superior and inferior vena cava are simultaneously ligated. The venous return to the right atrium is completely cut off. The empty atrium shows diastolic dilatation reaching its peak in the first two to three beats immediately following ligation and slowly decreasing to a flat curve within a few seconds. The experiment records the maximum diastolic negative pressure of –24 mmHg. The diastolic dilatation of the empty atrium establishes that the diastole is a reflex dynamic stretching of the atrial muscle fibers for the first time.

the canine went into cardiac arrest. We were unable to repeat this particular experiment on the same canine either because of cardiac arrest or because the canine remained in atrial fibrillation following the initial experiment. It was impossible to interpret the ongoing events during this particular experiment. The graphic tracing of events and atrial pressure changes were continuously recorded for further in-depth analysis and interpretation. We recorded the following observations. When the total venous return to the right atria was suddenly stopped the immediate response became apparent within the first three beats. When the venous return was stopped the graphic tracing increased to five times its original size and the atrium produced a negative pressure to –24 mmHg. This astonishing finding revealed for the first time that the atrium was capable of producing a remarkable negative pressure depending upon the venous return and thus indicating it could exert a very strong suction force during diastole. This suction force was of a potential and intermittent nature. However, this negative pressure was unsustainable for a longer period of time in this experimental model because of the sharp fall in blood pressure. Each result indicated cardiac arrhythmia and arrest.

We developed the following experimental model in which the venous return was suddenly and totally cut off but at the same time cardiac output was maintained by alternate means. This experimental model is explained in Experiment IV (Figure 8.4) done in one canine. This experiment had the canine at a 90° erect position. A glass jar (2,000 mL graduated cylinder; Kimble USA, Rockwood, TN) (Figure 8.4) was filled with Ringer's lactate solution and connected to the right atrium of the canine through an No. 18-French Silastic tube. The Silastic tube was connected to the right atrium through the inferior vena cava via a venotomy. Once the tube was inserted the venotomy was closed using a purse string of 3–0 silk suture to maintain a watertight opening. The Silastic tube was filled to the tip with the Ringer's lactate solution and clamped during insertion into the atrium to prevent an air embolism from forming. The Ringer's lactate level in the jar and the tip of the Silastic tube were maintained at the same level at the beginning of the experiment by maintaining the jar on a wooden stool of appropriate height. During this experiment both the superior and inferior vena cavas were clamped simultaneously, while the clamp on the Silastic tube was relaxed. We further observed the continuous passage of Ringer's lactate solution from the jar to the right atrium. We were able to continue this experimental model without the atria going into fibrillation. The flow of Ringer's lactate from the jar to the right atrium continued until the fluid level in the jar dropped to 5 cm below the original level, at which point the flow from the jar toward the atrium stopped. This established the limitation of the atrial suction force and demonstrated how the pressure gradient enabled the fluid to flow against gravitational force. We were able to immediately repeat the experiment in the same canine by raising the jar manually and returning the level of Ringer's lactate to its original level. We were unable to continue repetition of the experiment after a few trials because of a sharp fluid overload and cardiac failure.

Experiment IV.

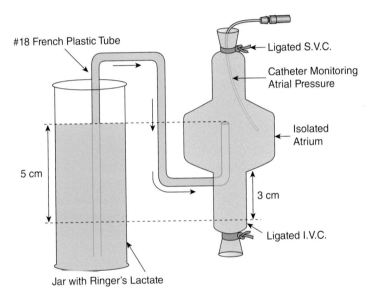

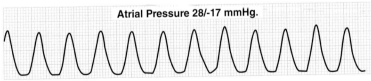

Figure 8.4 Experiment IV. The superior and inferior vena cavas are ligated. The right atrium is connected to a glass jar filled with Ringer's lactate solution through a no. 18 F size Silastic tube. The atrial diastole produces a suction force up to –17 mmHg, suctioning the solution from the jar during each diastolic expansion until the level of the solution within the jar reaches 5 cm below the original level.

Discussion

In the last chapter on the discovery of the motion of venous valves we are able to time the opening of the venous valves to the exact segment in the EKG recording and thereby associate it with a particular part of the cardiac cycle. We observed that the valves begin to open immediately after the blinking light followed by the QRS complex or after the ventricular systole and before the beginning of the P-waves before the atrial systole and coinciding with the atrial diastole.

Several questions were raised. What causes valvular motion? Is it a primary or secondary event? Since it is rhythmic with the heart what is its connection to the heart?

Following our experimental findings in a canine heart we can interpret that atrial diastolic dilatation of muscle fibers is an active phenomenon (see Experiment II). It creates negative pressure by suctioning blood from the inferior vena cava into its empty chamber. This triggers the motion of the blood column in the entire venous tree and the venous valves open passively. During systole of the atrium the chamber collapses onto itself and negative pressure is lost. Thus the suctioning function ceases. Due to gravitational force, which is of diametrically opposing the atrial diastolic suction force, the entire column of blood in the venous tree tends to flow in the opposite direction (i.e. downward toward the feet). As the venous valves are "one-way" doors opening toward the heart, the weight of the column of blood flowing downward closes the valves. Therefore during each cardiac cycle venous valve cusps open during atrial diastole and close during systole. Atrial diastolic suction force is related to the volume of venous blood return. Hence this force can vary during different positions of the body and is related to the variation of gravitational force. Although the motion of venous valves is present in all positions it is the least obvious in a supine position and is at its maximum in the upright position since it is in this position that gravitational force is at its peak. It was precisely for this reason that the experimental models were created in the unique upright positions.

A review of the literature shows that the maximum negative diastolic pressure ever recorded in a canine's right atrium is −4 mmHg. In healthy humans the minimum right atrial diastolic pressure ever recorded is 0 mmHg. Guyton explains that very close to the tricuspid valve a pressure of –2 mmHg can be recorded as a result of the downward motion of the valves during ventricular systole. This does not provide any functional significance.

In Experiment II by clamping the superior vena cava the venous return to the atria is partially cut off and its effect is immediately reflected in the graphic tracing. The height of the graphic curve (anachronic and dicrotic notches) increases remarkably and the negative pressure falls to –14 mmHg. This is a significant change in the negative pressure, that is, seven times lower than the resting pressure recorded in the experimental model in the recumbent position. This can be produced only by an extra dilatation by corresponding dynamic stretching of the atrial muscle fibers during diastole. In turn, this results in a more forcible collapse of the atrium during systole, increasing the positive force to 24 mmHg. This is noticed only for a few beats due to the clamping of the inferior vena cava, thereby causing a decrease in venous return and it results in a sudden fall in cardiac output. As a consequence arterial pressure begins to fall rapidly and within a few seconds the experiment had to be stopped.

In Experiment III the entire venous return to the atrium was cut off by simultaneously ligating the superior and inferior vena cavas. The effects of this experiment were interpreted by an evaluation of the graphic tracing and recording of the atrial pressure. Within seconds the arterial pressure reached a level that was not recordable and the experimental model's heart went into cardiac arrest following cardiac arrhythmia.

During this experiment the lowest atrial pressure recorded was –24 mmHg. Immediately following ligation of both vena cavas the graphic tracing indicated the highest graphic curve during the first three beats progressively falling to a flat line within 10 to 12 beats. The atria reached peak dilatation during diastole during the first three beats indicating its maximum reaction to the lowest venous return.

Starling's laws of muscle contraction state that the law of the heart is thus the same as the law of muscular tissue. Since then it is a common belief that systole is an active contraction and diastole is a resting period of the heart.[11] By these experiments we have established that this is not true for atrial muscle fibers which contract during systole and stretch during diastole. Starling's law of muscle contraction that is related to cardiac muscle fibers definitely needs modification as both contraction and dilatation are active phenomena of the heart. An empty right atrium records few beats of maximum diastolic stretching of its muscle fibers. Thus this is the reason why it produces maximum negative pressure by maximum stretching of its muscle fibers even when the venous return is completely cut off. This proves for the first time that the diastole of the atrium is related to active stretching of the muscle fibers. It is a conscious stretching of its muscle fibers as it reacts according to venous return. It also disproves our age-old thinking that diastolic distension is simply caused by the venous filling of the chamber. The corollary of this is that if there happens to be no venous return then the atrial chamber would remain a collapsed bag. This is similar to that of a collapsed pillow cover when the pillow is removed from within. This experiment also establishes the fact that the atrial chambers react to venous return and are capable of changing the negative pressure to exert the maximum suction force when venous return fails. The negative pressure reaches its maximum force when the venous return falls to its lowest level. It cannot sustain this action for a long period of time as this experiment is not compatible with life as total venous return is cut off during the experiment. So we developed the next model. Experiment IV was conducted in canines at 90° erect posture. The venous return is cut off by simultaneously ligating the superior and inferior vena cavas at the same time as the clamp on the Silastic tube is released, the atrial suction force is adequate enough to suck the Ringer's lactate solution from the jar. Thus, cardiac output can be maintained for a longer period of time without the immediate fall in arterial pressure. Graphic tracings demonstrate that sustained negative pressure exists. The Ringer's lactate solution continues to decrease until it reaches a level of 5 cm lower than that of the original level. The original level is exactly at the level of the tip of the catheter in the atrium. The reason why the passage of Ringer's lactate from the jar to the atrium stops upon falling to 5 cm below the original level establishes the fact that atrial suction force has limitations.

During this experiment we were able to maintain the canine model's arterial pressure for a longer period of time with steady graphic tracing when the negative pressure of the suction force in the atrium reached −17 mmHg. When the Ringer's lactate level fell below 5 cm of the original level the passage of fluid ceased. To continue this experiment we had to manually raise the entire jar to bring the level of Ringer's lactate to that of the tip of the Silastic tube in the atrium. It was possible to repeat this experiment in the same model. However, we could only repeat the experiment a few times because the cardiopulmonary system became overloaded with Ringer's lactate in a short period of time.

Conclusion

Atrial chambers have a dynamic function. They are not passive chambers and are not collecting tanks of venous blood as presently has been thought. The atrial chambers are strong suction machines dictating the venous return to the heart. This is the main force in the body creating motion of venous blood in the venous tree. Suction force is exerted intermittently during each diastolic expansion of the atria. This suction force is converted to a continuous pump owing to the presence of venous valve cusps. The venous valve cusps can open only in one direction, thereby maintaining venous blood continuously in motion in one direction toward the heart.

The four chambers of the heart have separate functions. Ventricles are forward pushing pumps. The left ventricle propels blood into the systemic arteries and the right ventricle pushes blood into the pulmonary arteries. The right atrium draws blood toward the heart from the systemic veins while the left atrium similarly draws blood from the pulmonary veins. In systemic venous circulation contraction of skeletal muscles and quiet respiration act as adjunctive forces assisting the motion of venous blood.

In summary, this article reveals through experimental evidence the following four discoveries:

1. The human heart is a dual machine forward pushing ventricles and backward suctioning atria.
2. The diastolic phenomenon of the heart is due to active stretching of its muscle fibers.
3. Cardiac muscle of all the four chambers actively contracts and dilates. There is no resting phase.
4. Venous valves in humans open and close during each cardiac cycle and are related to atrial diastole.[17]

chapter nine

Theory of circulation by the author

Concepts of the circulatory system

Concepts of the circulatory system evolved from the time of Hippocrates. This evolution spans almost two millennia until the appearance of Sir William Harvey. Harvey brought by his experimental work a complete overhaul of all the old teachings. He provided new doctrines that modern medicine follows today with mild modifications. Dedicated and serious indulgences of many other scholars and great minds contributed to this evolution and many of their discoveries are still held as the icons of modern medicine and with great reverence. However, these new concepts as an improvisation over age old concepts came in tidbits and at astonishingly prolonged intervals over several decades and even hundreds of years in some instances. Nevertheless, the practice of medicine has continued since the time of Hippocrates under the guidance of their concepts, even as we practice contemporary medicine today.

Preceding the time of Sir William Harvey, a period of which was close to 2,000 years, it was thought that the liver was the main organ of circulation within the human body. Retrospectively, this seems to be inconceivable and astonishing in view of our present knowledge. However, it was the belief of physicians during that era.

Prior to the Galen era the circulation of blood was thought to be only in the venous system. Blood was not thought to circulate in the arterial system since both the venous and arterial systems were considered separate.

There was not much change to earlier concepts with the exception that Galen entertained the idea that there is blood present in the arteries that leaked through the interventricular pores to the left ventricle. But their main function was that they carried the pneuma and the vital spirits to all the tissues and organs. Galen's

DOI: 10.1201/b22792-9

teachings and concepts remained as unquestioned doctrines of the theory of circulation for the next 1,500 years and were even practiced after the time of Harvey.

It was Harvey who established by experimental means that the left ventricular systole is the only force that circulates the blood through the arteries into the veins and back to the right ventricle. The right ventricular systole transverses the blood back to the left ventricle through the lungs. As a result of Harvey's experiments the human heart took center stage in the role of the circulatory system and achieved the status of the central organ of the body. However, one wonders why Sir William Harvey did not attempt to describe the role of the atrial chambers. He had a genuine reason to forego the role or importance of the atria as part of the heart and this deserves a detailed explanation and needs to be understood by the readers.

For a student of medicine at Padua University the main curriculum of the time was the study of philosophy, anatomy, and physiology as held by Aristotle and Galen. Naturally Harvey considered them his mentors and held them in great esteem. He particularly cites the name of Aristotle many times with reference to the anatomy of the heart in the last chapter of his book *Di Mortu Cordis*. Harvey also gave credit to Hippocrates as the first to recognize the heart as a muscular organ. Aristotle's concept is that the heart consists of two ventricles and the right and left auricles (the Latin meaning "ears") are just the remnants of the ventricles, as the auricles structurally resemble the ventricles, and thus their description. The concept of the atria as constituting two separate chambers of the heart was not explained. The atria were considered to be the terminal portion of the vena cava on the right side and the pulmonary veins named as the arteria venosa on the left side. Both were considered to be draining blood directly into the corresponding ventricles and were guarded by strong cone-like valves. Harvey inherited this anatomical teaching from his predecessors and continued to embrace the same views. In addition, Harvey explains in the last chapter of his book that "there are 3 forked portals in the entry of the vena cava and arteria venosa, lest that when the blood is most driven out by means ventricular systole, it should fall back ... meaning leak back to these veins." It is very evident that he accepted these large veins that were directly connected to the respective ventricles guarded by the tricuspid valves on the right side and the bicuspid valves on the left. Harvey, like his predecessors, did not appreciate the atria as separate chambers and as an essential part of the human heart. It was subsequent anatomists who clearly explained the heart as a four-chambered organ consisting of two atria and two ventricles. The auricles are part of the atrial chambers and resemble the ventricles in their muscular texture. The concept that the functioning part of the heart only consists of the ventricles and atria and are nonfunctional and passive chambers collecting blood pools of the heart is continued until today.

Classification of circulation

In reviewing the history of circulation, the experimental work of this author and the new concepts that are revealed approximately 400 years after the work of Harvey become important to review and understand. It is important to note that the circulation of blood takes place within a closed system. But the forces that keep the blood in motion are entirely different in the arterial and venous system. Under the credence of the findings described in this book we can classify circulation into four systems: systemic arterial, systemic venous, pulmonary arterial, and pulmonary venous. Each chamber of the heart is responsible for the motion of blood in its system; therefore the motion of blood in the systemic venous system is a result of the right atrial diastole and the pulmonary venous system is due to the left atrial diastole. The motion of blood in the systemic arterial system is caused by left ventricular systole and the pulmonary arterial system is caused by the right ventricular systole.

Until the present time only two chambers, the ventricles, are given credit for the motion of blood. Accordingly, this author brings a paradigm shift to our understanding of the circulation of blood in the human body. This does not contradict what has been documented and discovered by William Harvey on ventricular function. The work of the author complements and completes our understanding of the motion of blood in the human body, both in the arterial and venous systems approximately 2,500 years after its evolution.

In the arterial system motion of blood depends on the forward pushing forces that originate by the two ventricular systoles. In the venous system motion is dependent upon the suction force that originates in the atrial diastole. All four chambers of the human heart have a mechanical function and equally contribute to the circulation of blood in the human body. The heart is a forward pushing and backward sucking dual pump organ of the body (Figure 9.1).

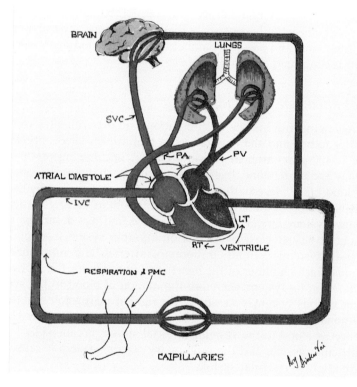

Figure 9.1 Theory of circulation by the author: PA = pulmonary artery; PV = pulmonary vein; SVC = superior vena cava; IVC = inferior vena cava. The right atrial diastole is the main force of systemic venous circulation, RES & pmc = respiration and peripheral muscular contraction. The left atrial diastole is the main force for pulmonary venous return. In the arterial system the motion of blood depends on forward pushing forces that originate in the two ventricular systoles. In the venous system the motion dependence is on the suction force that originates in the atrial diastole. All four chambers have mechanical function and equally contribute to the circulation of blood in the human body. In addition in the systemic venous system atrial diastole, peripheral muscular contraction, and respiration are the adjunctive forces.

The author has recorded in this book a few discoveries and novel concepts that I hope will serve as the foundation for the future understanding of the motion of blood in the circulatory system. The cardiac role doubles in its contribution and in its importance.

New insights

These discoveries did not take place in a chronological pattern. This author has narrated how it began with an accidental finding and how in the process of solving the jigsaw puzzle I stumbled upon the area of the heart. There were no overnight revelations. It took a very long time. The initial collection of data was done in small pieces taking a substantial amount of time to put them together and to interpret them.

The preparation of and embarking on experiments in the canine heart were a very promising beginning but the outcome of the experiment was not only not exciting but sometimes very depressing. After each experiment I took a considerable time off to reflect and embark on the next experiment. During each experiment events occurred so fast that there was no time to witness and interpret the findings during the experiment. There were many times during the experiments that the canine heart went into atrial fibrillation. Continuation of the experiment at that point was futile after an entire day of elaborate preparation of the model in the canine laboratory. Therefore after each experiment I would walk out of the canine lab with a sense of disappointment since I saw no light at the end of the tunnel with the exception of all the data collected and recorded. It is with these bundles of data that I walked out with a heavy heart. As I recovered I would review the data in detail, providing me with rays of light and enlightening my spirits. It took a long time for me to understand the secrets of atrial diastole that were recorded in the graphic changes and slowly being revealed. Ultimately it was a paradigm shift that I had to make in my own understanding of the cardiac muscle which contracts in the systole and stretches and dilates in the diastole. This paradigm shift opened the door to the mystery that both the systole and diastole are equally active phenomena of the heart.

After a long period of contemplation and reflection, a few years later I realized that there is no resting phase of the heart. As a matter of fact, there is no resting phase in the universal phenomena at all. Rest is a feeling of comfort and a word devised to explain a feeling experienced by the human mind. In reality it is a change of motion and rest is the experience of that change. The systole and diastole are both equally active phenomena with a change of motion. There is no resting phase for the heart; if at all there, it is that humanly unnoticeable pause that occurs between each systole and diastole when consumption of energy is at its lowest by the cardiac muscles.

The big jump I made was to get myself out of the box I was in, probably built around the doctrines of the great Professor Ernest Henry Starling (1866–1927), who was the most respected physiologist of his time. His doctrines were established upon the basis of experiments on the frog's thigh muscle and included that muscles contract and function in moving the joints.[11] When the muscle recoils back into its stretched state it is considered to be in the resting phase. These laws were established on striated skeletal muscles that are under the voluntary control of the somatic nervous system. We have since then unconsciously applied the same laws to the involuntary striated muscle fibers of the heart. Once I freed my thoughts that had been inculcated by the inherited teaching of many generations atrial function became very vivid to me and I was able to interpret my experimental findings with clarity and renewed confidence. It was clear that the atrial diastole is also an active phenomenon like the systole of the heart and equally contributes to the function of the heart. Thus we have recorded in this book the following new findings derived from the basis of a series of experiments that were conducted on the canine heart model and the data collected. We have also relied on the findings of the venous valvular motion recorded while performing descending phlebography in the human venous circulatory system:

1. Atrial diastole is an active phenomenon and functions like a suction machine of the human heart. It keeps the blood in motion in the systemic and pulmonary venous systems. Peripheral muscle contraction, famously labeled as the peripheral heart of the human body, and respiration supplement as adjunctive forces.
2. Venous flow of the blood is pulsatile as it relates to atrial diastole. It is subtle and very well noted in the central veins surrounding the atrial chambers.

3. Venous valves open and close during each cardiac cycle and are secondary to atrial diastole.
4. The function of the atrium is to keep blood in motion in the venous system at an optimal velocity and it is important to the maintenance of the "milieu interior" of the body like other parameters of the human body.
5. The cardiac muscles contract and stretch. Both are active phenomena with physical, chemical, and electrical changes occurring in each state.

References

1. Fabricius H. Ab Acquapendente. *De Venarum Ostiolis*. Padua, 1603.
2. Whitteridge G. *William Harvey and the Circulation of Blood*. American Elsevier, London/New York, 1971;115.
3. Aird WC. Discovery of the cardiovascular system: from Galen to William Harvey. *J Thromb Haemost*. 2011:9(suppl 1):118–129.
4. Harvey W. *De Motu Cordis*. The Classics of Medicine Library, Birmingham, Alabama, 1978.
5. *The Aphorisms of Hippocrates* (1561). Classics of Medicine Library, Birmingham, Alabama, 1982.
6. Grant R. Antyllus and his medical works. *Bull Hist Med*. 1960;34:154.
7. Wilson Leonard G. Erasistratus, Galen and the Pneuma. *Bull Hist Med*. 1958;33:4; 293–314.
8. Estienne C. *De Dissectione Partium Corporis Humani*. Simon de Coline, Paris, 1545;182–357.
9. Scultetas AK, Villavicencio JL, Rich NN. Facts and fiction surrounding the discovery of the venous valves. *J Vas Surg*. 2001;33(2): 435–441.
10. Sylvan T. Percutaneous retrograde phlebography of the leg. *Acta Radiol*. 1951;36:66–80.
11. Linton RR. The communicating veins of the lower leg and the operative technique for their ligation. *Ann Surg*. 1953;138:415.
12. Trendelenburg F. Uber die underbindunger vena saphena magna bei underschen-kelvarizen. *Bruns Beitr Klin Chir*. 1890;7:195.
13. Rai DB. Descending venography: venous approaches. *Proceedings of the 12th Annual Congress of the Phlebology Society of America*. 1989:58–64.
14. Kistner RL. Surgical repair of the incompetent femoral vein valve. *Arch Surg*. 1975;110:1336–1142.
15. Rai DB, Lerner R. Chronic venous insufficiency disease and etiology: a new technique for vein valve transplantation. *Int Surg*. 1991;76:176–178.
16. Rai DB. Phlebography. In: *Textbook of Angiology*. Chang JB, Olsen ER, Prasad K, Sumpio BE, eds. Springer Verlag, New York, 2000;1093–1100.
17. Rai DB. The motion of venous valves in humans—a new discovery. *Int J Angiol*. 2006;15:141–145.
18. Lurie F, Kistner RL, Eklof B. The mechanism of venous valve closure in normal physiologic condition. *J Vasc Surg*. 2002;35:713–717.

19. Gottlob R, May R. Function of venous valves. In: *Venous Valves.* Springer Verlag, Wein/New York, 1986;62–77.

20. Starling HE. *The Linacre Lecture on the Law of the Heart.* Longmans Grune and Company, London, 1918;22.

21. Rai DB. The dynamic function of the atrial diastole of the heart and motion of venous valves in humans. *Int J Angiol.* 2013:22;37–44.

22. Harvey W. *On the Motion of Heart and Blood in Animals (De Motu Cordis).* Gateway editions, 6073. H. Regnery Company, Chicago, IL, 1962.

23. Guyton AC. *Venous Valves and the Venous Pump.* 6th ed. W.B. Saunders Company, Philadelphia, PA, 1981;227.

24. Bollinger A, Rutishauser W, Mahler F, Grüntzig A. Dynamics of return flow from the femoral vein [in German]. *Z Kreislaufforsch.* 1970;59(11):963–971.

25. Guyton AC. Venous system and its role in the circulation. *Mod Concepts Cardiovasc Dis.* 1958;27:483–487.

26. Brecher GA. *Venous Return.* Grune and Stratton Company, New York, 1956;2.

27. Houssay BA. Pressure changes in the heart. In: *Houssay's Textbook of Human Physiology.* 2nd ed. McGraw-Hill, New York, 1955;105–111.

28. Saunders JB. Dec M. *The History of Venous Valves.* MTP Press, England, 1978;23.

29. Hansoti RC, Dharani JB. *An Introduction to Electrocardiography.* Kothari Medical Publications, India, 1973.

30. Raju S, Walter W, May C. Measurement of ambulatory venous pressure and column interruption duration in normal volunteers. *J Vas Surg Venous Lymphat Disord.* 2019;8(1):127–136.

31. Taheri SA, Pendergast D, Lazar E, et al. Continuous ambulatory venous pressure for diagnosis of venous insufficiency: preliminary report. *Am J Surg.* 1982;150(2):203–206.

32. Rai DB. Chronic venous insufficiency disease: its etiology and treatment. In: *Textbook of Angiology.* Chang JB, Olsen ER, Prasad K, Sumpio BE, eds. Springer Verlag, New York, 2000;1089.

Index

Note: Locators in *italics* represent figures and **bold** indicate tables in the text.

A

ABI, *see* Ankle brachial index
Angiography, 35, 38, 53
"Animal spirit," 7, 10
Ankle brachial index (ABI), 35, 38, 41
Aquapendente, *see* Fabricius, H.
Aristotle, 1
  age-old theories of circulation, 17
  anatomical structure of heart, 3–4, 16, 76
  experiments of heart, 2–3
  four temperaments, concept of, 7
  heart, three-chambered organ, 2
  qualities of human body, 1–2
  theory of medicine, 1–2
Arterial diastole, 15
Arterial pulse, *13*, 14, 45
Arteries; *see also* Circulation; Heart
  closed circuit, 19, 62
  end vessels, 4, 9
  femoral and tibial, 38
  flow of blood, 2, 13, 14, 20–21, 28, 31, 45–46, 63, 76
  pneuma, 2, 9, 12
  pulsation of, 16–17, 45–46
  systemic or pulmonary, 31, 73
  and veins, connection between, 15
  vital spirit, 2, 4, 12, 13
Auricles or ears, 16, 20, 76–77

B

Black bile, 6, *7*
Blood, 6, *7*
  atria, storage house, 4
  circulation of, *see* Circulation
  flow in arteries, 2, 6, 7, 13, 14, 20–21, 28, 31, 45–46, 63, 76
  flow in venous system, *see* Venous blood flow
  functions of, 62
Bloodletting, 4, 6, 9, 14, 28
Blood pressure, 32–34
  sphygmomanometer, 31–33
Boyle, Robert, 19, 27–28
Brain, 3, 4, 7

C

Cadaver dissections, 1
Canines
  continuous and simultaneous recording of monitors, 64, *65*
  EKG monitoring, 47, *48*, 64, *65*
  experiments, 63–69
  heart, experimental model, 60, 61
  mongrel, 27, 47, 63
  position of canine, 65–66, *66*
  study on, 63–69
  superior and inferior vena cava, 65–69, *67*, *69*

Cardiac arrest, 43, 67, 68, 69, 71
Cardiac failure, 69
Chronic venous insufficiency disease
    (CVID), 32, 34, 38, 39, 42
Chronic venous ulcers, 51
Circulation
    age-old theories of, 17
    arterial limb of, 43
    of blood, 30, 75, 79
    classification of, 77–79, *78*
    closed-circuit system, 62
    concepts of, 75–77
    "ebb and flow" theory, 29
    gamma curve, *38*
    history of
        impact, 8–10
        phases of, 1
    respiration, role of, 63
    theory of
        by author, 75–81, *78*
        concepts of circulatory system,
            75–77
        galenic era, 4–8, *7*
        by Harvey, 14–15, 19–21
        pre-galenic era, 1–4, *5*
        at present, 24
    venous, 24, 25, 27, 41, 46, 57, 73,
        78, 80
Colombo, Realdo, 6
CVID, *see* Chronic venous
    insufficiency disease

D

Deep venous thrombosis (DVT), 35,
    40, 42
*"De Mortu Cordis and De Circulatione
    Sanguinis"* (Harvey), 18
Descending phlebography, technique
    of, 52
Diastole
    arterial, 15
    atrial
        canine's heart, experimental
            model, 61
        description, 63
        discussion, 70–73
        dynamic function of, 61–63

rhythmic opening and closing
    of venous valves, 61
study on canines, 63–69
dilatation or filling (resting) phase,
    45, 46
DVT, *see* Deep venous thrombosis

E

Ebb and flow theory, 6
EKG tracings, *see* Electrocardiography
Electrocardiography (EKG tracings),
    47, *48*, 49
Erasistratus, 1, 29
Estienne, Charles
    De Dissectionne Partium Corporis
        Humani, 29

F

Fabricius, H., 11, 12, 14, 17, 29, 46
    theory of circulation of blood,
        11

G

Galen, Claudius, 1
    "animal spirit," 7, 10
    background, 4–5
    circulation, theory of
        galenic era, 4–8, *7*
        pre-galenic era, 2–4, *5*
    doctrines of circulation, 12–14
    ebb and flow theory, 6
    four humors and temperaments, 2
    function of venous valves,
        discovery of, 28
    teaching and practice of medicine,
        18
Galileo, 11

H

Hales, Stephen, 33
    blood pressure, 33
Hardcopy recording, 47
Harvey, William
    background, 11–12

efforts on ventricular chambers, 4
experimental revelation of, 14–15
experiments with ligatures, *13*
methods, 12–14
revolutionary discoveries, 9
theory of circulation, 14–15, 19–21, *20*
   anastomosis between arteries and veins, 14
   auricles or "ears," 20
   future generations, 21
   types of ligatures (tourniquets) on arm, *13*, 14
ventricular function of heart, 15–19
   age-old theories of circulation, 17
   anatomy of heart, 15–16
   diastole, 18
   discovery of valvular function, 17
   forward pushing pump mechanism of ventricular systole, 20–21
   systolic contraction of ventricles, 16–17
Heart; *see also* Circulation
anatomical structure of, 3
atrial diastole
   canine's heart, experimental model, 61
   description, 63
   discussion, 70–73
   dynamic function of, 61–63
   rhythmic opening and closing of venous valves, 61
   study on canines, 63–69
defined, 3
as first organ formation in body (Aristotle), 2
as four-chambered organ, 3, 16
"a hot cauldron—blood warming pot" (Galen), 6
Herophillius, 1
Hippocrates, 1, 6, 12, 28, 53, 55, 58, 75–76
Human Physiology (Houssay), 63
Humors, 2, 6, 7, 8, 9

L

Ligatures (tourniquets) on arm (Harvey), *13*, 14
   softer ligature, *13*, 14
   tight ligature, *13*, 14
Liver
   animal spirits, 10
   blood flow, 2–3
   circulation in body, 7, 8, 75
   to express love and emotional feeling, in Arabic, 8
   origination of veins, 2
   as sanctum sanctorum of love, 8
   transformation of food into blood, 4, 5, 62
Lungs
   capillaries, discovery of (Malpighi), 14
   functions of blood, 62
   pneuma, 6, 9
   vena cava, ascending portion, 3–4, 7, 12

M

Malpighi, Marcello
   discovery of capillaries in lungs, 14
Modern medicine, 11, 75
   history of, 51, 62
"Mogul" emperors of India, 8

O

Orleans, Cailiuse, 29
   existence of venous valves, 29

P

"Peripheral heart of the body", *see* Venous circulation
Phlegm, 6, 7
Plato, 1
"Plethora and Plenitude", 29
Pneuma (air), 2, 4, 6, 7, 8, 12, 75
Post-thrombotic syndromes, 51, 58
Praxagoras, 1, 2
Pulsation, 16–17, 18, 45, 46

R

Rai, D. B.
    personal experience, 52–53
    reflection, 58–60
    theory of circulation, 75–81, *78*
    using balloon catheter, 52

S

Seldinger Technique, 53
"STRIP TEST," 12
Systole
    active contraction, 46, 71, 80
    atrial, 49, 70–71
    contraction of heart or vessels,
        45, 46
    ventricular, 15–16, 18, *20*, 21, 23, 27,
        30, 31, 45–47, 58, 63, 71, 76–77

T

Temperaments, 2, 7
Trendelenburg, Frederick Adolph, 51
    etiology of varicose veins, 51

V

Valvuloplasty or valve transplant,
    52, 58
Varicose veins, 51, 58
Veins; *see also* Circulation
    arterial, 18–19
    distal, 12, *13*, 14
    end vessels, 9
    femoral, 25, 35, 38, 52, 53, 54, *55*,
        56, 61
    hepatic (portal), 4, *5*, 6
    ipsilateral iliac, 36, 37, *37*, 38, 39, *39*
    jugular, 53, 54, 64
    motion of blood, 12, 25, 31, 46, 62
    origination of, 2
    popliteal, 56
    pulmonary, 3, 10, 15–16, *20*, 24,
        31, 76
    superficial, 11–12, 39
    systemic, 31, 73
    varicose, 51, 58

Vein valve transplantation
    below knee, 32
    surgery, 12, 34, 39, 42, 52
Venorum Ostioles, 29
Venous blood flow
    arterial pressure, 42–43
    arterial pulse, 45
    circulation time, 39, 41–42
    contraction of heart or vessels
        (systole), 45, 46
    deep venous thrombosis, 42
    dilatation or filling (resting) phase
        (diastole), 45, 46
    findings, 48–41
        chronic venous insufficiency
            disease, 38–39
        circulation time, 38, *38*, *39*, *40*
        deep venous thrombosis, **34**,
            39–41, *40*
        pre- and post-operative studies,
            40, 41, *41*
    intermediary phase, 46
    materials, 34–35
    method
        electrocardiography (EKG
            tracings), 47, *48*, 49
        gamma camera, 34, 36, 37
        hardcopy recording, 47
        semi-recumbent position, 35, *36*
        time activity curve, 36, *37*
    objective, 34
    pulsation, 45
    velocity, 31–33
    venous valvular incompetency,
        41–42
    ventricular systole, 45
Venous circulation, *24*, 25, 27, 41, 46,
    57, 73, *78*
Venous insufficiency, 51, 52
Venous valves
    history, 29–30
    in humans, motion of
        author's personal experience,
            52–53
        author's reflection, 58–60
        discussion, 55–57
        exposure and frame number,
            54, *55*, *56*, *57*

history of modern medicine, 51
management of venous
disorders, 52
methods, 53–54
results, 54–55
mystery of, 27–29
circulation of blood, 27
laws of muscle contraction, 27
Venous valvular incompetency (VVI),
38, 39, *40*, 41–42, 52

Ventricles, 3, 16–20, 56, 62–63, 73,
76–77
Vital spirits, 2, 4, 6, *7*, 9–10, 12, 75
VVI, *see* Venous valvular
incompetency

Y

Yellow bile, 6, *7*